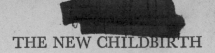

THE NEW CHILDBIRTH

There is no doubt that the birth of her child is one of the most important moments in a woman's life, and the excitement of this moment can be destroyed by the accompanying pain and dread which have come to be accepted in our society as inevitable.

But this pain and dread can be controlled. Childbirth is a natural function and anguish can give way to triumph.

Erna Wright is a pioneer of this method of controlled childbirth, which is already widely accepted; and here is a precise account of her system in book form. The necessary physical training is explained in detail, sufficiently clearly to provide both a text book for doctors and midwives and a handbook for expectant mothers. *The New Childbirth* is undoubtedly the most important advance in midwifery to date, and is a standard work on the subject.

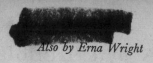

Also by Erna Wright

THE NEW CHILDHOOD
PERIODS WITHOUT PAIN

THE NEW CHILDBIRTH

Erna Wright

With a foreword by
Elliot E. Philipp, F.R.C.S., F.R.C.O.G.

A STAR BOOK

published by
the Paperback Division of
W. H. ALLEN & Co. Ltd

A Star Book
Published by Universal Tandem Publishing Co. Ltd, 1964
Revised Edition 1965, reprinted 1966, 1967
Second Revised Edition 1967, Reprinted 1968
Revised Edition 1968, reprinted 1969 (twice), 1970 (twice), 1971 (twice),
1972 (twice), 1973 (twice), 1977 (twice), 1978

This edition reprinted 1979 (three times),
by the Paperback Division of
W. H. Allen & Co. Ltd
A Howard & Wyndham Company
44 Hill St, London W1X 8LB

ISBN 0 352 30475 8

Made and printed in Great Britain by
Hunt Barnard Printing Ltd., Aylesbury, Bucks.

For the Mothers and Fathers
who are
the Roots of our Society.

ACKNOWLEDGEMENTS

The author would like to express her appreciation to Gillian Bayens for the drawings, Christopher Mason for the diagrams, Anne Obermer for the lecture transcripts, Dorothy Smith for typing the manuscript and Sarah Charles for editing and compiling the book. Thanks are also due to John Minshall for supplying the photographs.

Contents

Foreword

by Elliot E. Philipp, F.R.C.S., F.R.C.O.G.

ERNA WRIGHT has written an excellent book. This is not surprising to those who know her; for her qualities and experience are unique among the many people now attracted to the practice of psychoprophylaxis in obstetrics.

As the book explains, psychoprophylaxis is a relatively new system of preparation for childbirth. It involves the elimination of some old fears and old ideas, and substitutes new information, new techniques. These techniques are quite easy to learn; in class their constant repetition in the company of others turns them into habits; they are then reproduced in labour, for which the mothers are thoroughly rehearsed by the system.

In other words, it is a form of coaching for labour. Like any other handbook or text-book, it reinforces the coaching, or partially substitutes for it when no coach is available. It also teaches the elements to those who, by virtue of their training as midwives, doctors or auxiliaries, wish to have at their side an easily absorbable résumé of the practice of psychoprophylaxis, to help *them* help their patients during pregnancy or labour.

What are the qualities that make Mrs. Wright an ideal person to write this book? She is a big personality. There is nothing small and nothing petty about her. She is the devoted mother of three healthy, well-balanced, happy children. She has more sense of practical humanity than most people—more even than many of those who devote their lives to looking after others. Because of her happy and contented home life, she can be an active pioneer, filled with almost missionary zeal, who yet never becomes hard or bitter if others try to thwart or contradict her. Unlike most missionaries, she can retreat home, for there her husband understands and helps her enormously.

Her experience is wide and she is a fully-trained nurse. At first she trained individual mothers privately in the system, which she was learning by trips abroad, by reading, by talking and corresponding with others interested and, above all, by watching and helping women in labour. Soon the demands on her time became so great that private lessons had to stop; then she taught only in classes—with the advantage that mothers of all social groups could learn together from one another as well as from their teacher. All spoke a new language in a new way—and the "old wives' tales" were eliminated.

Then came the day when she was asked to organise psychoprophylactic training for midwives, doctors, students and patients in an important teaching hospital—in fact, one of London's leading hospitals.

This book is the essence of Mrs. Wright's teaching; it is a notable advance in British midwifery. It is a privilege to be asked to write the foreword to what is certain to become the standard handbook on the subject in the English language.

Introduction

I HAVE written this book for two main groups of people.

First, those expectant parents who have heard about this new method of preparation for childbirth, but live too far away from anyone who can teach it. For these parents, this book, if used exactly, and with the approval of their doctor or midwife, can form a reliable preparation for perhaps the most exciting event in family life. Both mother and father will know exactly what to expect and will know all the words which are used by doctors and midwives in "labour-ward jargon".

Most important they will both know all the things which each can do to assist the birth-process. For the first time in our culture, expectant parents can know that they need not be helpless in the face of the birth of their child, but can be partners in the team which ensures the safe arrival of the new member of the family.

The second group of people who will, I hope, find this book useful, are midwives, health-visitors and physiotherapists who are concerned with expectant mothers. Many of my friends and colleagues in this field of work have asked me to write a hand-book which they could keep for reference.

In the busy life we lead, for those who work to help others, time is precious and limited. Therefore the teaching of new ideas had to be in a highly concentrated form; bits and tips are often crowded out by other necessary information. This book offers this second group of readers the step-by-step "recipe" for ante-natal preparation according to the principles of psychoprophylaxis. All the small details have been carefully included.

I hope almost nothing in the following pages will be

found too controversial in the light of modern obstetric practice. My dearest wish would be fulfilled if midwives worked together with their patients, following the training through, and thus were partners in this exciting adventure—active parenthood.

Perhaps both groups of readers would care to know a little about the background to this method and how it came to print through my hands. My own first experience of childbirth led me to seek a way of making birth an experience to be looked forward to rather than dreaded. I discovered the teaching of Dr. Grantly Dick Read, once considered to be so revolutionary, and approved of his ideas on the possibility of joy instead of fear. I was one of the small percentage of people for whom his teaching worked exactly as "The book said". But I found that unfortunately it often led to misconstruction and therefore to disappointment, both for mothers and midwives.

It was this experience which led me to want to make my success available for other women by ante-natal teaching. As soon as I began to teach I discovered the flaws. The vast majority of women were grateful to be enlightened about childbirth—an experience about which no one would talk openly. All they had to go on were vague reassurances that "everything will be fine, we will take care of you", from their doctors and from their friends, encouraging statements like, "You wait until the pains start, then you'll know what life is all about".

Caught between these two forms of exquisite torture, millions of women have endured needless emotional and physical suffering for too long. So I should like to pay a very sincere tribute, as just one of millions of grateful women, to Dr. Grantly Dick Read, as the first medical practitioner with the courage and enlightenment to fight this evil tradition and replace it with clear, simple information. Perhaps his greatest contribution lies in the fact that he was the first pioneer and took on his shoulders all the burdens and all the brickbats. We who followed him, however different our approach might be, have good reason to thank him.

The mothers of today who have only vaguely heard his name, and who meet the ever-increasing number of enlightened doctors and midwives who are willing to encourage their efforts to learn, should know that it was he who laid the foundation of such enlightenment in the western world.

However, Dr. Dick Read's practical teaching was not sufficiently advanced to give adequate physical help to the majority of women and my results were disappointing. But they led me to a quest for something better.

I found it in Paris in the spring of 1960. Dr. Pierre Vellay, a follower of Dr. Fernand Lamaze, offered me his work with the most open-handed generosity. His staff of teachers gave up what little free time they had to teach me. His patients allowed me to watch them during preparation and in labour. They taught me, too, by sharing their thoughts with me during the birth of their babies; they did this with delight, knowing that in my presence with them lay the chance to make the kind of experience they were having possible for British women too.

On my return to London, I began to use what I had learnt with my first group of mothers. Although the ideas I was cautiously expressing were new here, the results soon caused a stir of interest among doctors and midwives as well as among pregnant women. There was no lack of opposition either. But the great majority of workers in the ante-natal field expressed approval and enthusiasm, once they had cared for patients who had been trained according to the new approach. Many have come since then to learn for themselves, so that they too can carry these benefits to an ever increasing number of their patients. Some hospitals—including one London teaching-hospital—are offering this new approach to their patients under the National Health Service. Several Local Authorities have even paid the fees for their staff to be trained in this new method.

If I tried to list all the individuals and organisations, interested in caring for the people of tomorrow, who have given their time, money, and encouragement in an effort to help me to "spread the word", the list would be longer than this book . . . I only wish I could thank everyone personally and individually. All I can do is to hope that they will accept this book as my personal expression of thanks for their contributions, without which I would have been unable to develop this approach.

The words may be mine; but the work—and this book—are their gifts.

October 1964   ERNA WRIGHT

Lesson 1

WHAT THIS BOOK IS ALL ABOUT

THIS book is about something called "psychoprophylaxis".

Psychoprophylaxis is a made-up word which literally means "mind-prevention". So this will indicate that it has something to do with people but not especially with childbirth. Actually the basic approach has been used successfully by dental patients and people in many other "stress" situations.

Applied to childbirth the teaching falls into two main categories. First, education so that the mental background is suitable as a basis on which to build physical preparation; then the physical training. The method originated in Russia, where the first mother "trained" in the psychoprophylactic sense gave birth to her baby in 1949. A French obstetrician, Dr. Lamaze, learned the principles from his Russian colleagues and adapted them for use in the French cultural situation; his first successful patient gave birth to her baby in 1952.

Since then, great strides have been made in the development of the method in many countries: South America, China, and—since the official approval of the late Pope Pius XII—Italy, Belgium, Spain and Portugal. The method can be used basically, by *every* expectant mother; different levels of education, intelligence, and background make no practical difference to the possibility of success. Each woman takes from the course of training what she is able to digest and use. Therefore for each woman, that which she takes is sufficient. Each woman needs only one qualification: she must be willing to *work* conscientiously towards the birth of her baby.

The majority of women in each country have similar cultural backgrounds so that although the method has been adapted in each country to fit that background, the principles have not been changed. For instance, in Europe we use sectional diagrams as teaching-aids, while Chinese teachers find that they need full-size plaster models of everything. (These models, by the way, are exquisitely lifelike and the models of the new-born baby would appeal universally to any woman.) Even the breathing techniques have been slightly adapted to fit the majority of women in different countries. Foreign women who live in Britain and who have so far made use of this training have not found any difficulties of language and custom which they could not overcome by a little diligence and intelligent co-operation between them, their teachers, and the medical team who assisted at the birth.

A "trained mother" in the psychoprophylactic sense means a woman who has been educated to understand the way her body works with particular reference to the working of nerves, muscles and the reproductive system. She understands that childbirth is (usually) a normal function of her body—but she understands, too, that bodies do not always behave as they ought and that doctors and midwives are trained to observe them in labour and to apply special measures if normal functioning does not take place. A trained mother has some knowledge of what differences may occur in labour if it is not normal, and knows how to adapt herself to such different situations. Long before the actual birth of her baby she understands the reason behind the ante-natal check-ups. She understands why everyone emphasises the importance of correct diet and rest. After all, good medicine is simply common sense applied to a specialised field.

What can a "trained" mother hope to accomplish? From the labour reports sent to me by my ex-pupils, it would seem that 35% of them have experienced a *painless* labour. Not a sensation-less labour because any body-experience will result in some sensations; but a labour during which none of the sensations, however strong, were interpreted as pain by the woman herself.

There are several factors needed to accomplish the experience of a painless labour. Excellent physical health and a perfect position for the baby inside the womb are natural requirements. The bone structure of the mother must be of adequate size. Her attitude towards the experience of the birth of her baby must be in perspective. She should not expect to lie and think beautiful thoughts and hope that the baby will appear as if by magic. If she had such ideas, she would be bound to be disappointed and pain and fear and confusion would occur.

Conversely, the mother who is convinced that suffering is inevitable has also got things all confused, and neither extreme of attitude would help any woman to be in the 35% group. BUT . . . a healthy optimism, based on the firm knowledge that one has done everything possible to prepare oneself and that one is ready to do one's best—this is a vital factor.

. Lastly, the approval by doctor and midwife of the preparation has considerable positive influence. Even if doctor and midwife are not familiar with this particular method, yet understand and agree with the principle of self-help in labour, their attitude assists the woman to maintain control.

You will no doubt say: "Yes but how about me? I'm not the sort who wins prizes as a rule and my premium-bonds have never come up either." "What if I *do* have pain during labour?" Yes, I am even more interested in you. You are in the 65% majority—the women who will, for one reason or another, experience pain, or at least discomfort, during their labour. The reasons might be physical or emotional. This is not important. What matters is: how about you?

. Again, I quote reports from my pupils. "I had pain during the latter part of my labour and the doctor said it was because . . . but as long as I carried on doing what you had taught me to do, I remained in control. The pain never overwhelmed me." This is a representative phrase which has been repeated over and over again by those who were in the 65% category.

In other words, a trained woman cannot "fail". There is nothing in which to fail. She knows that all she needs to do is handle her sensations exactly as she has been taught; then she can remain in control; of course her husband and the team who are with her during labour may need to help her to reinforce her control.

Terms like "success" or "failure" are meaningless. Women don't go into labour as an endurance-test or an obstacle-race. But they *can* go into labour armed with a valuable means of remaining on top of their own experience.

Therefore any woman with common sense can be trained so that she herself becomes a most useful and co-operative member of the obstetric team which watches over her own, and her baby's well-being, before and during the birth. During the birth, she uses correct breathing and specialised training of muscle-control in relationship to the work her body does, and uses them automatically. This physical activity, based on knowledge, enables her to become a skilled accompanist who enhances and supports the automatic function of labour. Clinically this will lead to a generally more efficient labour. Often this is shorter than it might otherwise have been; but even if—for reasons outside anyone's control—it isn't, the physical strain of the total happening is still visibly lessened and recovery is faster. If we only take the narrow clinical view, this in itself might be enough reason for expending additional energy of both mothers and teachers to accomplish the training.

However the effect of psychoprophylactic preparation goes much further. When you think about it, only some 30% of labour is the physical aspect; the other 70% is the emotional and psychological experience for the mother. It is in this field that psychoprophylaxis really comes into its own. We have already received many letters—over 4000 of them—which say: "Thank you for making the birth of my baby possible, while I remained a dignified human being in control of my own reactions." These speak for themselves; but midwives and doctors too have confirmed what they say, again and again. They have described the obvious delight their patients have shown, not only after birth but during labour. And they have been infused with renewed enthusiasm by the controlled approach their patients used in the handling of their physical processes.

If all or any of the above holds any interest for you who read it, I hope you will read on. If you are a couple expecting the birth of your baby within the next few months, you might like to start by reading through all the lessons. Then at about four months pregnancy, begin with the exercises which are part of Lesson 1. Then add the others—but don't start these until 26 weeks pregnancy. You will find instructions as you go along, to discontinue some exercises and to add others. Carry out the instructions as exactly as you can.

If you were attending psychoprophylactic classes you would meet a new chapter of knowledge in each class and new exercises to add to the ones you have already learnt. You use this book in the same way—especially if you re-read each lesson as you come to the exercises which accompany it.

The lessons are based on the classes my expectant mothers receive, and contain the same information, in the same order as they have it in class. You will find learning easier if you choose a day to make your "class day" each week, and if you take up the next lesson on the same day each week. In between, you should practise the exercises you have already learnt—but only *once* each day. It is important not to become exhausted when practising and not to have too much to do all at once. There is no value in practising exercises ten times, because there is a limit to how much your brain and nervous system can absorb in a given time.

Learning how to give birth is like learning any other skill—learning to ride a bicycle, drive a car, play a musical instrument, operate a knitting-machine or indeed learning to read and write for that matter. All the many things we all do almost automatically have been learned in this way; this is the built in learning-mechanism human beings have. Physical skills are learnt with mechanical effort and precision, practised in small "lumps" and then gradually become almost automatic. Any time that we are awake we can drive, ride, write, read and so on. So it is with the skill of giving birth and doing so with control and with dignity.

Go over the lectures which accompany each lesson several times and look at the drawings carefully so that you become familiar with all the things you will meet during your pregnancy and particularly during labour. If your husband is willing, his help with the later exercises and his understanding of the chapter "The Necessary Father" will make the whole experience of training and birth a memorable one for *both* of you. Incidentally there is nothing in this book which *any* human being should not read. My own teenage daughter has heard my recorded lectures many times and is eagerly looking forward to being able to put this teaching into practice when she expects her first child. My two younger children have seen the diagrams and photographs; their only reaction has been a sense of excited wonder at the fascinating and beautiful events which form part of our development.

I should like to think that you, the expectant parents who read this book, will form a "class" which spans the British Isles. Before you begin, however, make up your mind to follow one "recipe" for preparation only. There are many methods and many books have been written. The greatest disservice you can do yourselves is to attempt to "mix your drinks". If you do it with alcohol, confusion results. The same thing happens when you mix ideas.

If you are a professional reader, and hope to use this book in the preparation of your patients, the above principles obviously apply equally. Modified application will produce modified results. You will find a list of useful teaching-aids and the names and addresses of suppliers at the end of the book in a special index. There is also a film mentioned in the index which can be borrowed as indicated, by professional users who teach classes of expectant mothers. I can only hope that your work with this material will bring you the same thrills and joys which I have already been privileged to experience.

Most readers, however, can probably be divided roughly into three categories—like the women who come to my classes. First, there are those who come because a friend recommended them. They have been told "She works you terribly hard, but having a baby afterwards is so much easier so you don't mind the hard work". Starting on that basis, you might possibly be in quite a muddle, not knowing exactly what we are doing; you probably believe all sorts of things which you would discover are not true. And you would also find that some of the things you believe *are* true.

Then there are the people who have read *everything*—and the amount of literature which is available on how to have a baby is quite formidable! Textbooks, leaflets, pamphlets in red, blue or pink. If you have done this, as I did, you will probably by now suffer from a healthy state of mental indigestion. For instance, there is one book written by a psychiatrist which simply takes every known method of preparation for childbirth existing on this planet—and there are 33 of them—and describes each one without comparing them! That is to say, the writer doesn't tell you whether this method yields more than that one, he simply *describes* each one. And after reading each one you think "this is it"—until you turn the page and find another, practically the same except that there is far more difficulty! When you finish the book, and it has something like 890 pages, you feel like screaming.

If you are in this state, you at least ought to know that we don't use all 33 different methods! We use just one; you have already read a brief description of what we do.

The third category contains those of you who find expecting a first baby (or a second baby) frankly frightening. Now let's face it, this is not a crime. It is hardly surprising that you are frightened of having a baby—if all the propaganda hasn't passed you by. And as you begin to look even vaguely pregnant the propaganda won't pass you by—those women "out there" will see to it that it doesn't. So if you have become even a little affected by this disease called "having a baby", then it's time we helped you to make up your own mind whether having a baby is really something to be frightened about.

The first lesson explains quite simply all about what we are going to do. If you look at the index on page 7, you will see that every week you learn a little more, both in terms of information—things you have to know in order to have a baby efficiently—and in terms of what to do. And by Lesson 8 the picture will be completed.

Now, before you can learn—and this is the most important part—what you do during the birth when it happens, you have to make sure that the tools you are going to use are fit for the job. And the tools you are going to use to do whatever-it-is are the muscles of your own body. Fortunately, you don't need special instruments and you don't need gadgets of one sort or another; you've got your own gadgets and instruments right there. So the first few exercises will be concerned with your gadgets, the muscles which you're going to use in one way or another during labour. You will find these on pages 30, 31, 32, 33, 34, 35, 36 and 37.

This is excellent for forty to forty-one weeks—about the

length of your pregnancy. But then there comes the point when the baby is ready to emerge from its "nursery" inside the womb, when it is ready to take up independent life. Here comes the most delicate question of all: how to get out of there? Of course, there could be all sorts of ways of getting out of "there"—up through the stomach, chest and mouth, for instance. But we don't have a technique for delivering babies this way. Really the only practical way is down through the bottom of the pelvic basin. This is why we are so concerned and interested in making the muscles in this area of the body stretch adequately, with ease, and not with difficulty—with difficulty any old muscles will stretch—and then regain their original elasticity. When you are thinking of muscles, think in terms of the elastic that holds up your panties because basically they're very similar. Good elastic, as you know, will stretch to accommodate a bulging waistline, but still retain its elasticity. So what we must do, among other things, is to get the muscles of the pelvic floor to do the same.

Now when we talk about the baby coming out through the opening in the pelvic floor, you might be wondering, particularly if this is your first baby, just how big *is* this baby which is going to come out of there? The standard British baby in 1960 weighed 6½ lbs., was 20 inches long and the circumference of its head was 14 inches—these are the statistical averages. So this is roughly the size of the baby which is going to emerge from your pelvis. But it is not spreadeagled all over the place. It is nicely folded, packed like a fold-away fridge or a fold-away washing-machine, so that it occupies the least possible amount of space, as economically as possible. So this is the first comforting fact you might like to remember!

A reminder about remembering:

You may have already discovered, and if you haven't, then you will as your pregnancy advances, that one of the side effects of pregnancy is what is called *maternal amnesia.*

Gradually you become less and less capable of concentrating on anything except your thoughts of yourself and your baby. And you will find this particularly hard—if you haven't already—if you are normally alive to current trends, if you are with it. Whether it's pop songs or the political situation doesn't seem to matter. I have known girls of seventeen who were pregnant, who just adored a particular star or group, yet three weeks before the baby was due, their idols would be on television in the room next door and they wouldn't move because they were finishing a sock! That sort of thing just didn't matter any more. Or you will perhaps have found, or will find in the future, that if you decide, say, to go to the kitchen and fetch something, when you get into the kitchen you will have completely forgotten what it was you went for. Have you noticed this? Perhaps you can't even remember whether you have! Memory is distinctly affected by the hormones which are produced by the body in pregnancy. This is quite normal and it wears off, so you can return to your interests later.

But it might mean you have to make a bit more effort with these lessons and exercises. Perhaps it would help to make notes in a special notebook, just a child's exercise book, bought specially for the purpose. Or you can use the special blank pages provided at the end of the book. But don't worry if it takes a bit more time and trouble than you expect. And remember, as I said earlier, any skill worth learning *does* demand effort.

Practical 1

NEW MUSCLES AT WORK—AND
CONSCIOUS CONTROLLED BREATHING

WHEN you begin to learn and practise the exercises in this book, you should remember that each one has a special purpose which is explained as clearly as possible. If you are very rushed on any one day, it would be better not to practise on that day but to leave it until you are fresh again. But don't do this as a regular habit, because your nervous system can only develop skills with regular and frequent practice.

You should do your exercises on the floor rather than on your bed—a bed is usually too comfortable and you cannot feel the exact sensation in your muscles if your mattress supports you too well. However, you do need to be comfortable, so collect as many cushions and pillows as you need for this purpose. The diagram labelled "1" shows your basic position. Adopt this for the exercises, but vary the number of pillows under your head and shoulders to your own needs.

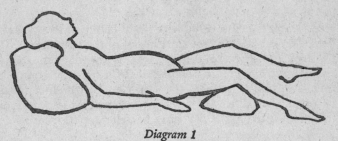

Diagram 1

First, let's find out where your "gadgets"—the muscles you must learn how to use—all are. If you look at Diagram 2 (overleaf) you will see an odd shape which is a picture of a

part of the bony framework of your body which is called
the PELVIS. It consists of two identical bones at the sides
called the *innominate bones* or "nameless" bones; these are
joined by a triangular bone called the *sacrum,* at the back.
The pelvic bones meet in front to form the *pubic arch.* You
might run your hands over some of the landmarks of your
pelvis so that you know exactly where we are working. If
you stand with your hands on your hips, your palms touch
the upper ridges of the bones of your pelvis. Run your
forefinger down from your navel along your tummy and
you will notice that the elastic tummy becomes a hard bony

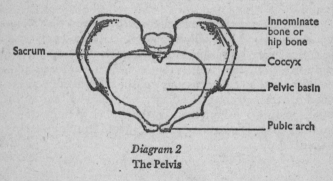

Diagram 2
The Pelvis

area, which is well covered with flesh. This hard bony area is
the point where the two large bones of the pelvis meet, to
form a kind of keystone above what is known as the *pubic
arch.* If you stand with your legs slightly apart and run your
finger up one leg, across the lower end of the bony area
between, then down the other leg, you will get some idea of
this arch—although it can only be felt properly during an
internal examination.

If you lie down on the floor in the basic position "1", you
will notice that the flat bone in your lower back soon feels
uncomfortable. This is the *sacrum,* and it needs a small
pillow to support it in comfort, particularly during preg-

nancy when the shape of your body changes. Attached to the sacrum like a little tail are five tiny bones, all fused together. These are called the *coccyx*. The coccyx is all that remains in the human body of a tail. All these bones and associated muscles are known as the PELVIC BASIN.

It helps to know these "official" names, for they are all words which you will hear when you go to the ante-natal clinic, and to know them will give you a rough idea of what people are talking about.

Now why are we so interested in this pelvic basin? Well, for both men and women, the organs of reproduction are contained in the area of the pelvic basin. But the male pelvic basin is narrower and more triangular than the female one—which is much more basin-shaped. This is important, for you will see from Diagram 3 that in the middle of the female pelvic basin is the WOMB—or UTERUS, which is the official word you'll keep on hearing during your pregnancy.

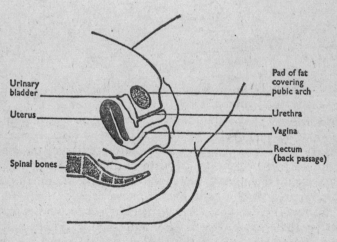

Urinary
bladder

Uterus

Spinal bones

Pad of fat
covering
pubic arch

Urethra

Vagina

Rectum
(back passage)

Diagram 3
Contents of Pelvic Basin

This uterus is the nursery where your baby lives until he has grown sufficiently to live independently, when he is born. The uterus is about the size of a pear when a woman is not pregnant; but after about 12 weeks of pregnancy it is already so big that it overspills from the pelvic basin into the ABDOMEN or tummy. It continues to grow as the baby grows and it is this growth which gives a pregnant woman her characteristic shape. Wouldn't it be useful if your flat could grow in the same way? I am sure you will appreciate, from your experience in the kitchen, that any basin must have a bottom in order to be of use. Without a bottom to a basin the contents would fall out, whether rice or gravy or whatever; so it is with the pelvic basin. But although the

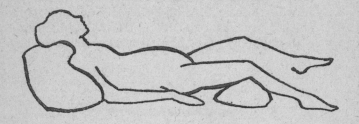

pelvic basin is made of bone all round, the bottom is not. It is made of a hammock of strong muscle—and by the way, when we talk about muscle we mean what is commonly called FLESH, whether it covers arms or face or pelvis. These pelvic muscles at the bottom of the basin will come into play during the actual birth of the baby. So we must make sure that they are as supple as possible, and many of the exercises you will be practising are done for this purpose. Incidentally, this hammock of pelvic muscles isn't called the bottom. The medical profession is terribly polite and they don't call anything the bottom of anything. So they—and we—refer to it as the PELVIC FLOOR.

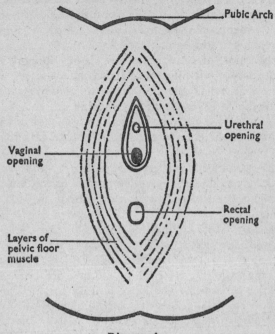

Diagram 4
The Pelvic floor, as seen from outside

Before doing the exercises, we must know how to do them properly. Whenever we make our body do any work which is more than the usual amount—and this is what exercise really means—the muscles use more body-fuel, which is stored from our food. To do this efficiently they need more OXYGEN. Oxygen is a gas which is present in the air, more so in fresh than in stale air, so always do your exercises in a room with an open window. The amount of oxygen we take in by ordinary automatic breathing is not quite sufficient for doing extra work so under such circumstances we feel our body demanding more. Think

back to the last time you ran after a bus. You will recall that
when you reached it and collapsed into the nearest seat you
were probably puffing a bit—the body's way of saying
"more oxygen and faster please!"

This is not, of course, the best way of doing it. It is far
better to recognise the need in advance and provide the
extra oxygen by adapting one's breathing to the work one is
making the body do. We do this by using

CONSCIOUS CONTROLLED BREATHING

This is something every athlete learns—and from one
point of view, labour *is* an athletic performance. Most of the
exercises we do in preparation for labour are also in this
category.

The first level of conscious controlled breathing will be
used with this first set of exercises and the others we need
for labour will be added gradually. Always do the controlled
breathing with a steady rhythm and take great care to keep
it regular and exact. The more you watch this the better
your control will be. *Level 1.* Lie in the basic position. Take
a breath in through your nose with the lips closed. If you
push your shoulders back against the pillows you will feel
your chest fill comfortably, but not excessively. Then blow
the breath out through your mouth as though you were
blowing on a spoonful of hot soup. Breathing in can be done
in a fairly leisurely way, but the blow out should be crisper.
Notice when you breathe in, how your bosom is lifted up,
and how it sags when you blow out. You will feel a little pull
from your tummy-muscles when you do Level A breathing,
but the effort should be made with the chest muscles.
Practise the breathing for about half a minute and try to get
about *six* breaths in and out into that time. Never hold your
breath and don't stop in the middle. Just keep the rhythm
and rate steady.

Now combine this breathing with the following limbering-up exercises. Take the breath *in* during the first half of each exercise, and *blow* during the second half.

LIMBERING-UP EXERCISES

(a) Lift one leg keeping the knee straight, as high as you can with comfort, while you breathe in. Drop the leg back to the resting position while you blow. Repeat with the other leg.

(b) Lift one leg slightly off the bolster and swing it out sideways without tilting your hips. Swing the leg back to rest and repeat with the other leg.

(c) Grasp one ankle on the inside with the same hand (right ankle—right hand). Breathe in and push the knee towards the floor until you feel a stretching sensation on the inner surface of the thigh. Blow as you return the leg to rest. Repeat with the other leg.

(d) Lift one leg just off the bolster and turn the leg outwards. Rotate the foot six times and return to rest. Repeat with the other leg.

Note: Rotation should be done clockwise with the right leg and anticlockwise with the left leg.

PLEASE NOTE that each of the above is to be practised *once a day*. This also applies to all the other exercises. Do take care to time the beginning of each exercise with the beginning of the controlled breath as this gives you good practice for what you will do later during "labour rehearsals" and during labour itself.

Next we shall find out what work the muscles actually do. All muscles work in the same way. When they perform the work for which they are designed, the threads or fibres which make up a muscle shorten and thicken. Examine the muscles of your hand when you make a fist, and you will see this very clearly. The greater the amount of work demanded of the muscle, the shorter the fibres become. We call this action the CONTRACTION of the muscles. Muscles do not actually contract individually but in groups. So when, for instance, you squeeze your face into a tight grimace, the group of face-muscles all contract together.

The uterus is basically a group of muscles and it works by contraction also. Since we are preparing to work with the uterus during labour we must be interested in the way in which its work happens. Now some muscles contract when we want them to; but there are others which do their work independently of our will. The important difference between the face-muscles, for example, and the uterus is that the face muscles work when we want them to and the uterus works independently.

Now we know what happens when a group of muscles works. But what happens when it rests? The fibres lengthen and become thinner again. In the case of muscles which we control by an act of will, we undo the contraction when we wish. We call this *decontraction* of the muscle, which results in RELAXATION.

Our next exercise is the drill to give us practice in becoming aware of the sensations which come from a group of muscles in a state of contraction and how they feel in a state of relaxation after we have decontracted them.

And we must also learn how to do this with the muscles of the pelvic floor. We use these muscles all the time, without realising it, so the exercise is not too difficult. Whenever we go to the toilet, these muscles come into play. Contracting the pelvic floor simply means that you tighten the buttocks and the lower tummy-muscles, and then contract the muscles you use when you feel the need to go to the toilet, but it is inconvenient to do so at that moment. Do this slowly; contract first around the back passage (rectum) and then around the front passage (vagina and urethra). Then decontract them, and notice what this feels like.

ACTIVE DECONTRACTION DRILL

Lie in the same position as for limbering up exercises. Using Level 1 breathing, breathe in, contract all the muscles of the left arm. Check exactly what this feels like. Blow out and at the same time decontract the muscles of the arm. Repeat, using:-

> Right arm.
> Left leg.
> Right leg.
> Muscles of pelvic floor.
> Upper chest and shoulder muscles.
> Face.

This is how you learn to control individual groups of muscles. With practice the sensations will become quite clear to you. You should stay mentally alert and be aware of what you are doing. This will condition you to recognise instantly when any group of muscles is in a state of contraction however slight. Do this drill once daily.

After you have done the active decontraction drill, check that none of the muscles you have worked with have inadvertently contracted while you were doing something else. If they have done so, then correct them. After about two minutes of checking in this way, the exercise is completed.

Now you will be in a lovely relaxed state—but there is no point in staying that way! You cannot do so in labour for any great length of time. So now prepare the body for activity once more. As the whole action-rate of the body has been slowed down by this exercise, we must *gradually* increase it, otherwise you may feel giddy or faint. Never jump up suddenly after this decontraction-drill, but clench and unclench your hands and wiggle your feet a few times before you s-l-o-w-l-y get up.

GETTING UP. Usually when we have been lying down we raise our bodies by using our tummy muscles. But this is

3

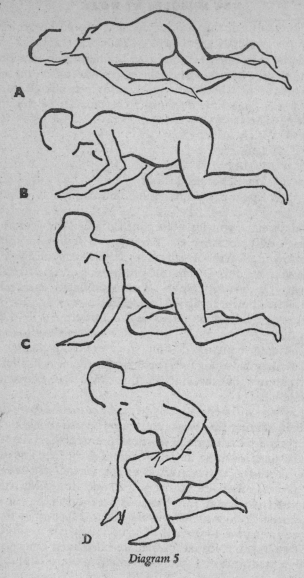

A

B

C

D

Diagram 5

too strenuous during pregnancy, and should be avoided. This rule applies to getting up after exercises, getting up from the bath and getting up from bed. Instead, this is what you do: turn on your side, bringing your arm over with you. Raise yourself on to your hip, using the over-arm and hand to support you. Roll over on to your knees and then get up on to your feet one after the other. Do the whole exercise as s-l-o-w-l-y as you can—think of a slow motion film and you'll get the idea.

THE PELVIC ROCK. The last exercise for today is concerned with the way you stand and walk when you are pregnant. Go into your ante-natal clinic and watch the girls—they waddle like ducks, especially those who are getting towards the end of their pregnancy. To begin with, it looks terrible. Secondly, it puts the whole weight of the pregnant uterus and the baby on to the muscles of the back instead of distributing it equally between back and tummy-muscles. No wonder so many women complain of backache. It is often, if not by any means always, due to this waddle.

The exercise we are about to learn will strengthen the back-muscles and will teach you how to walk elegantly, even though you *are* pregnant.

Stand with your feet slightly apart and with the knees loose. Put the palm of one hand under your "bulge" and the other on to your sacrum. (This position of the hands is simply to help you feel at first what your muscles are doing during the exercise; they don't need to be there all the time.) The breathing is normal, not conscious controlled breathing. Now lift your "bulge" with the sling of muscles underneath and at the same time push your "tail" towards the floor. Release both groups of muscles and then repeat the exercise. If you are doing this correctly you will feel your pelvis rock like a cradle. Do the rock 6 times, two or three times a day—while waiting for a kettle to boil or standing to answer the phone. I wouldn't practise it in public, though: the wiggle will entertain the people in the

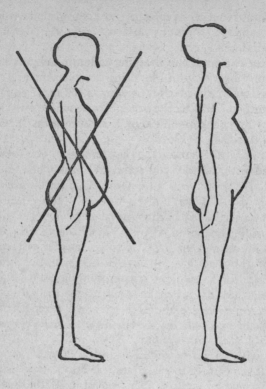

Diagram 6

bus-queue behind you far too much! This exercise is the strengthener. In addition, whenever you are walking, particularly when you are carrying a shopping bag, do *the first half of* the exercise and keep it that way. This means that you pull the bulge up and push the tail down and keep them in that position while you walk.

Do it in front of a mirror at first, and you will see how much more elegant you look and how much better your clothes look, too. Don't forget to keep your shoulders up—the exercise is impossible to do with rounded shoulders!

All these exercises will not take more than about 10-15 minutes per day. This will be enough until you begin the next exercises in about eight weeks time. But if you have only started on these exercises after the fifth month of your pregnancy, you can carry straight on next week with the exercises which follow Lesson 2. DON'T start lesson two until you are six months pregnant—so that the skills you learn from then onwards are fresh when you need them for the birth of your baby.

Lesson 2

THE DO'S AND DON'TS OF PREGNANCY

THERE is much controversy about the many aspects of keeping well and remaining in a state of comparative comfort during pregnancy. My lecture to mothers on this subject is constantly being amended as new products come on the market and mothers bring them to class to see if others might like to know about them and find out if I think they are useful. The following text is a finalisation of the latest information at the time of publication and later editions may well contain changes.

These are not rules but suggestions, which should help you to keep your well-meaning family—however well-meaning—at bay, letting you know at the same time what sort of ideas have helped many other women in the past.

I like to begin at the feet and work upwards. And this brings us to controversy No. 1—

SHOES. Do you or don't you wear high heels during pregnancy? The answer is YES if you have worn them before. Many girls have worn high heels since their early teens and the body has adapted to them. If they now go into flat shoes only because they are pregnant they may be very uncomfortable. The right approach is to wear the kind of shoes which are most comfortable at any given moment, and to change when you feel the need to.

There are various aches and pains to many women in pregnancy which can easily be avoided, but which unfortunately usually fall into the "What do you expect when you are having a baby?" category. Aching calf-muscles, swollen ankles, cramp in the feet and legs at night are of this type. All of these discomforts are usually due to venous dilation; this means that the blood vessels which carry blood back to the heart from the legs are not working as smoothly as usual, mainly due to the increased pressure of the pelvic organs. The answer is to be found in:-

STOCKINGS. Particularly in the articles called "support stockings". These are *not* the elastic stockings which you can get with a doctor's prescription, and which are only needed for varicose veins. Support stockings are made of nylon which has been elasticised and are hardly distinguishable from non-run nylons. They cost from £1.50 to £2 per pair; but two pairs will probably take you through the whole of your pregnancy as they don't ladder easily, if at all.

How do you use support-stockings correctly? You should choose them half a size larger than your usual stockings, and state whether you normally buy stockings of extra long leg-length. They come in many fashion-shades so you can choose a shade you like. (Don't put up with the first pair an assistant is trying to get rid of!) Keep your stockings and belt on a chair by your bed, so that you can reach them without getting out of bed. On getting up in the morning pull your stockings on while still sitting on your bed with your legs stretched out. Then swing your legs over on to the floor, pul your belt on and fasten your stockings. *Now* you can stand up and continue your morning routine.

Never stand or walk without your support stockings on, however short the distance. Don't let vanity tempt you to go out to parties in thin nylons—your comfort is far more important! Always have your bath at night and then go to bed immediately. Otherwise the veins will be unsupported again, and your efforts during the day will come to nothing. If you have to undress—at the clinic for instance—well, that can't be helped. Anyway, it's not very often. If you wear your support stockings religiously as I have indicated, it will be goodbye after about the first week to aches and cramps at night, and what a relief that will be! Of course they will feel rather hot in summer—but won't swollen ankles from the heat feel much worse?

These stockings are really only needed if you experience the discomforts I have indicated. They do apparently also offer some protection against varicose veins which seem imminent, but have not yet actually occurred. If the worst has happened, elastic stockings *will* be needed. These stockings are worn under ordinary nylons. Do take your doctor's prescription to a large shop which stocks them—the selection of colours will be better.

BELTS. From stockings to "what you keep them up with" is a logical step. If you wear support or elastic stockings, you will have to wear a maternity roll-on otherwise the stockings will pull the belt down. Maternity roll-ons have an inset where the "bulge" is and this expands with the bulge. You should add a third pair of suspenders to the lower edge for safety.

If all this is not necessary, an ordinary maternity suspender-belt is all you need, especially during the summer. Basically it consists of a piece of one-inch-wide elastic which fits under the "bulge" in front and over the hips at the back. The suspenders should be separate ones. As for maternity corsets—they went out with grandma!

You should always make sure that a belt isn't *too* well supporting. To check this, put it on, fasten your stockings to it, and then try to do the "pelvic rock" exercise while wearing it (see page 35). If you can do it, the belt will not prevent your muscles from working. If you can't do the exercise in it, hand the belt back to the Victoria and Albert Museum where it belongs. If you do need a special support belt for your individual case, your doctor will prescribe one.

BRAS DURING PREGNANCY. You may have already discovered that bras for pregnant women are not particularly well designed. What make should you buy and how do you know if it is correct for you? Any make of bra which is intended for support, and which has a cup with circular stitching so that there is no pressure on the nipple, is suitable. But a bra which merely consists of two cups with a fastening at the back is not suitable after about the first 12 weeks of pregnancy once the breasts begin to enlarge. So you may have to change bras two or three times during pregnancy depending on the rate of growth. Don't, however, throw bras away because they have become too small. You will find them useful after the baby is born and when weaning begins, for then you will notice the breasts becoming gradually smaller again. Cotton bras are healthier and more comfortable than nylon ones during pregnancy because cotton is more absorbent.

During the last four weeks before your baby is due you should wear a bra at night as well as by day. This is when the breasts need even more support and eight out of 24 hours without support is a long time.

Some women notice a slight discharge being secreted from the nipples during pregnancy. This is coloestrum—an early fore-runner of milk-production. If you think that the "leak" might come through on to your dress, fold a paper handkerchief into a pad about the size of the palm of your hand and put it in the lower half of the cup. This will absorb any secretion and can be thrown away and renewed frequently. But many women don't have this secretion indicating lactation, yet breastfeed very successfully nevertheless. So either way—don't worry.

NURSING BRAS. This is another hotly controversial subject. Hospitals ask you to bring two or three nursing bras in with you and they usually suggest that you buy them two sizes larger than your usual size. Well, I don't know who dreamed that idea up but it certainly isn't a very good one. The only satisfactory way to buy a nursing bra is to wait until the fourth day after the baby's birth and *then* measure the size of the bust.

This seems to indicate that your poor embarrassed husband will then have to go to a shop and choose a suitable bra . . . I cannot imagine anything my husband would care to do less. Answer? There is a type of nursing bra which we have found over the years to be good, and easily available. It unfastens with hooks and eyes in front and thus avoids the flap-cup which so often causes congestion in a full breast.

Having made sure of your supplier remember to take a tape-measure into hospital with you or to keep it handy at home if your baby is going to be born in your own home. For the first few days after the baby's birth you wear your end-of-pregnancy bras. The milk will come in—with a whoosh during the third day after the baby is born, and until the supply has settled down, a kind of make-shift suntop support, fashioned from a couple of nappies and a few large safety-pins will see you through. When the milk flow has become adjusted take the following measurements: (i) the width across the widest part of the bust over the nipples, including the back of the chest; (ii) the circumference of the chest immediately under the bust. These two measurements will indicate to the expert what size bra and what cup-size you need. Send these two measurements to your shop—and there you are. The little towelling pads you find in some bras are not much use. Again tissue hankies are much easier to deal with and much more hygienic, because you can change them so easily. The bra is called "MAVA"—see index.

YOUR SKIN IN PREGNANCY. By this I don't mean the skin on your face but on those parts which are stretching to accommodate tummy and bust bulges. You may have noticed that this stretching skin is becoming dry and itchy-a sure sign that it needs nourishment. What nourishment? Well, it *is* a large area! So facial creams which are expensive can only be used by the wives of millionaires. The rest of us need something much cheaper. Baby Oil, Nivea Oil or Cream, almond oil and liquid lanolin are all excellent. Olive oil stains underwear yellow and the stains can't be removed.

The simplest method of supplying it to the skin is the "lazy" way. Just add two tablespoons of oil to your daily bath and that will do beautifully. If you find this idea revolting, massage the oil or cream into the warm moist skin after your bath. You will not remain like a dressed lettuce-leaf, because your skin will absorb the oil greedily. Don't forget that the bust also suffers from stretched skin. While you are oiling, you might as well prepare your breasts for breast feeding—if this idea interest you. If you don't wish to breast-feed, ignore the next paragraph.

PREPARATION FOR BREAST FEEDING. Do this daily, please! Have a saucer of oil ready and oil the first two fingers and the thumb of one hand. Support the breast from underneath with the other hand and place your oiled fingers and thumb just above and below the areola (the brown area surrounding the nipple). Then with a smooth movement combined with pressure, guide the fingers and thumb forwards and slightly downwards over the nipple. Repeat this movement 4-6 times. And then treat the other breast in the same way. The oil will also prevent the coloestrum from sticking to the nipple and this makes it easier to wash off. You are actually imitating the action of the baby's mouth which the breasts will later experience. This massage of the breasts acts as a stimulation to lactation and helps the nipples to take on the correct shape for feeding.

INTERCOURSE DURING PREGNANCY. What a hush hush subject! We are still affected by a conspiracy of silence about it as the result of our Victorian and Puritan background. But people's natural urges are not limited just because no one dares to talk about them. During the first three months of pregnancy intercourse should usually be avoided on the days when a period would have been due if pregnancy had not occurred. The days when the *third* period would be due are particularly dangerous. On these days there is a risk of miscarriage. During the last four weeks of pregnancy intercourse should also stop. Here there is the risk of infection, with the secondary one of causing uterine contractions and possibly premature labour.

At all other times intercourse is all right. But you and your husband might try experimenting with different positions so that you need not feel uncomfortable.

After the baby is born, intercourse should be avoided for the six weeks before the post-natal check-up. Then you can be sure everything is back to normal and the delicate tissues have healed. Incidentally, the fact that you have not recommenced menstrual periods and the fact that you are breast-feeding are no guarantee whatever that you cannot conceive!

REST. This is perhaps your most important contribution to your own well being. And not only physical rest but mental "letting go" too. Your nervous system will help and this is why you will find that you are less and less interested in outside things. Don't kill yourself trying to prove that pregnancy doesn't interfere with your normal life.

It should interfere. Trying to do a full-time job, look after a husband and decorate the kitchen all at the same time is a foolish endeavour. It is equally mad to rush around cooking for numbers of friends whom you must entertain, or to stay up until the small hours. Your body will not put up with it and your doctor's raised eyebrows over your heightened blood-pressure will be your well-deserved punishment.

There *are* a few women who, in spite of the greatest care, still find that their body does not adapt well to its extra duties during pregnancy. These women are in a minority. Most of us can keep well with, among other factors, a few sensible rules concerning rest. How much rest? An hour after lunch—when you have stopped working away from home, this is easy—not necessarily asleep, but lying down with your feet up; you should be in bed by 10 p.m. watching T.V. or reading if going to sleep early is difficult. Let your mind as well as your body have a holiday. Reading light fiction is not a cultural crime, nor is watching T.V. serials, instead of working. Your emotions will be a bit topsy-turvy during your pregnancy and sudden changes from dejection to wild enthusiasm are very common. These changes are the result of hormone activity in your body and are a side effect so don't make them bigger than they are. Remember that a tired body reacts more strongly.

DIET. You may have found yourself crossly wondering "Why am I weighed *every* time I go for a check-up?" or "Just what are they trying to make me keep my weight down *for*?" The answer is simple: excess weight means excess strain on the body. Eating the correct things will help you to keep your weight within reasonable proportions. Again, there are a few women who need to gain more weight than they do. But they are a tiny minority and they will get detailed advice on what to do from their doctors. I am speaking to the *majority* of pregnant women—people like myself, who only have to think of sugar and pastries and our mouths water.

Don't worry about the baby. He will do nicely, thank you. His weight-gain is determined by heredity and the placenta (the organ on which he lives while he is in your womb) will take all he needs directly from your bloodstream—if necessary from your teeth and bones and hair. You don't want this: you want to be beautiful as well as healthy. You want to be able to wear a decent dress, too, after junior is born. So here is your answer: Keep your *own* check on your weight gain and counteract any occasional "sins" with stricter self-control afterwards. Actually it is very simple. You *can* eat anything and everything, you can eat and drink as much as you like ... *except* the foods which are officially called *carbohydrates*. Bread, potatoes, sugar, pastries, cake, chocolates, sweets and alcohol come into this category.

It is equally important not to cut out carbohydrates altogether. You *are* allowed the following *daily* quantity of carbohydrates: two slices of bread (the size of a large sliced loaf) or the equivalent in brown bread, crispbread or whatever fancy variation you favour and *one* medium sized potato. And remember, if you have a small portion of, say, rice or spaghetti, then this must come out of your carbohydrate ration, too.

Sweeten your drinks with saccharin-type sweeteners. Remember that glucose is just the same as sugar from the calorific point of view. You can season your food as you wish, including the use of salt.

Eggs, fish, cheese and meat—eat as much of these as you like. Liver is excellent, eat it every day—if you *can* eat it every day. You can eat cream and butter ad lib. too and they won't hurt you. But the sad thing is that you can't really eat them ad lib. without the carbohydrates to go with them. You know, a bottle of double cream can be a bit dull without the fruit salad, and the fruit salad contains syrup which of course contains a great deal of sugar. Sugar and starch, as far as your digestion is concerned, spell CAUTION: CARBOHYDRATE!

But *fresh* fruit—this is a very different matter. Fresh grated apple, pears, fresh grapes, oranges, cherries, bananas, peaches, apricots, strawberries, raspberries, melon, the delicious Chinese fruit called lychees—you can have a feast of these, and with as much cream on as you like. *But not sugar.*

You shouldn't have cornflakes or all-bran or porridge for breakfast, because you eat sugar with them. (Quite apart from the fact that cornflakes are also to some extent carbohydrates.) What you can have for breakfast on this diet is bacon and eggs. But only two pieces of toast, or of bread.

Is it alright to have cereal instead of the bread? Yes, you can swop. But you can't have a great big bowl with masses of sugar *and* some toast afterwards. And if you have marmalade or jam, that's even worse. The rule is: swop your carbohydrates around but *don't* have all of them together.

Now the question of milk. Milk contains the valuable commodity calcium. If you like milk—and some do and others don't—you can drink that famous pregnant women's pinta-a-day and that's about all. But if you hate milk, you needn't feel any longer that you are sinning against yourself and your child if you don't drink it. What you must do is to get your calcium in some other form. You get it in eggs, for example. But you'll get it much more effectively if you eat lots of cheese. Yoghourt is good, and the yoghourt is for some people much easier to eat. But go easy on the sugar when you have yoghourt, and stick to the natural unsweetened kind. The fruit-flavoured ones all contain sugar. And whether you cheat with honey or jam instead, it makes no difference—it's still sugar! You must have something with it but ... make your choice very carefully. Why not try fresh fruit?

You will want some measure, some standard by which you can judge whether you are overdoing it or not, in terms of food and in terms of weight. Remember that excess weight-gain makes the body work under unnecessary strain and can affect the filter of nourishment to the baby. But even if nothing worse than weight-gain occurs, this is still extremely difficult to get rid of after you have had the baby.

You can find out quite easily how you're getting on because the total weight-gain for an average-sized woman should be 24 lbs. throughout the whole pregnancy. But wait a minute ... People who are shorter than 5 ft. 3 ins. shouldn't put on more than 22 lbs. maximum. And people who are getting on towards 5 ft. 8 ins. or 6 ft. can go up to 28 lbs. with safety.

This does not mean that you must now eat all out, to put on that amount of weight. You don't need it. There are some people who put on 7 lbs. during the whole pregnancy and they're fine, and so is the baby. Don't try to push it up; try rather to keep it down. Watch yourself; if you put on approximately a pound a week and no more than a pound a week you'll be doing very well and you'll find that the rest evens itself out. By this I mean that if you are eating correctly, some weeks towards the end you probably won't put on anything. Fine—otherwise you would get more than your 22 to 28 lbs. You shouldn't put on more than approximately 4-4½ lbs. in a month to stay within your safe margin.

Well, you can hardly lapse into unconsciousness when you stand on the scales to be weighed—so you will know yourself, when you are sinning! Anyway if you *want* to look like an overgrown doughnut, that's up to you.

Still you may be—I hope you will be—invited out to dinner or to a party and if there is roast duck, roast potatoes and all the trimmings, followed by a fruit salad including everything with sugar and cream—for Heaven's sake, eat it! Enjoy it! This isn't an Association for Cruelty to Expectant Mothers.

But for the rest of the week be very conscientious. And this goes for alcohol, too. The odd drink (and I am assuming that none of my readers are secret alcoholics), the odd glass of sherry, a glass of wine with your dinner—these are fine. But if you're accustomed to drinking three cocktails before every meal and then a bottle of wine as well, then look out! Alcohol, remember, is converted sugar, and in quantity it has the same effect as bread and potatoes. Quite apart from rendering you somewhat incapable, you might fall and hurt yourself, but this is a secondary consideration. Alcohol, like starch and sugar, is fattening—so these are your enemies!

MORE MUSCLES AT WORK—AND MORE BREATHING

By now, you will have found that several things are getting much easier—that is, if you have done your best to practise with real concentration every day.

Mainly, you should have noticed that your awareness has become sharper of how muscles feel when you contract them and when they are at rest. Your ability to synchronise breathing with muscular activity will have improved somewhat.

But if the difference in the way your body responds when you practise, is still not very great, don't despair. These are early days yet and many people develop skills slowly. Just continue to practise daily. It will gradually become a matter of course to find your body doing what you want it to do.

Today's exercises are more numerous than those we learnt in Lesson 1. There are three for the muscles of the pelvis, and three which teach conscious controlled breathing in the extended form which will be needed for labour. But first of all, something more general:

Exercise 1. I am sure you will already have met those well-meaning people who tell you what you can and can't do about lifting things during pregnancy. Unfortunately they fall sharply into two groups, whose advice is quite contradictory. The "Lift-nothing-in-your-delicate-condition" merchants would have you spend the whole forty weeks of your pregnancy reclining on your bed. The other group say breezily, "Nonsense dear, childbirth is a natural function. Keep active—exercise is *good* for you!" For them you would have to drive a tractor on the day of your baby's birth, just to prove you're healthy! Both groups are only showing that they do not understand how the body works. The truth is, you can lift anything which you are normally capable of lifting without strain—*provided you adopt the right position for your body.*

So when lifting either a dropped hankie or a toddler, do it this way: Put one foot in front of your body and bend both knees as you go down towards the ground. When you lift both your body and the object, you will feel your thigh-muscles pulling the weight, instead of the muscles of your back and tummy.

Practise this a few times at first and you will soon do it naturally. Continue this habit after your baby is born. Teach it to your husband, too. Many men come into hospital with a hernia (or rupture) which is due to tummy muscles weakened by not lifting things off the ground correctly.

Exercise 2. Sit on the floor "tailor-fashion". If it feels hard, sit on a cushion but don't lean against anything—make your back-muscles support your body in an upright position. The exercise you are about to learn will help to increase the suppleness of the muscles of the pelvic floor. It is really an exercise taught and practised by all dancers. For our purpose though, it is done in reverse. This is because the reason dancers do it is exactly the opposite to ours; a dancer needs a tight pelvic floor but for labour we try to achieve the opposite.

Put the soles of your feet together, with heels as close to your body as possible, without losing your balance. Grasp your feet together with one hand and put the other hand *under* your knee. Now push the hand towards the floor with your leg and then bring the leg to its previous position with your hand. Notice that the muscles on the outer side of the thigh are pulling against the muscles on the inner side, which are called the *adductors*. Repeat, pushing towards the floor in one smooth movement and bring the knee back once more. After six repeats change hands and do the exercise six times with the other leg. Then keep your feet together without holding them and use both hands, under both knees simultaneously, again repeated six times. Don't jerk the knees downwards—just push as smoothly as possible each time.

After a few weeks of doing this whole pattern once daily, you will find that you can bring your heels closer to the body, without losing balance—the proof that your adductor muscles have lengthened, thus stretching the pelvic floor. (Post-natal exercises will reverse this again.)

Exercise 3. This has become a boon to many expectant mothers who suffer from backache. The exercise is intended to make the muscles covering the back of the pelvis more supple.

Kneel on the floor, sitting back on your heels. Rest your hands on the floor in front of you, with the elbows turned outwards and slightly bent. Put your head down and hump your back. Now, using your thigh-muscles like pistons, push your buttocks out backwards—like a duck lifting its tail. Feel your thigh-muscles doing the work. Then make them pull your buttocks back again, as though you were trying to hide them. Repeat six times.

Alternatively, you can do this exercise sitting on a hard chair about halfway along the seat. Plant your feet firmly on the floor in front of you. In this position, hold your thighs with your hands, to feel the muscles at work.

If ever you find that your back suddenly goes into a spasm, especially after bending down—don't stay in a bent position but sink on to your knees instead and do this exercise. After a few minutes the cramp-like sensation in your back will ease. This exercise is often beneficial also in early labour, if backache is experienced. It is then combined with the breathing-technique appropriate to that stage of labour.

Exercise 4. Once, in class, one expectant mother jokingly

remarked that this exercise was like "playing square bears". And this odd name has stuck to the exercise!

Kneel on the floor, with your knees slightly apart. Put your hands flat on the floor with your arms held straight. Your back should be arched slightly upwards, so that your body forms a square between knees and hands. (Like the position of a bear standing still.) Do the exercise as follows:

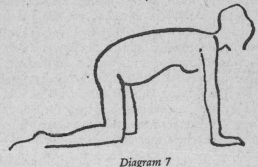

Diagram 7

Contract the muscles surrounding the back passage (anus)—decontract, repeat with muscles surrounding the front passage (urethra, vagina) and then the whole pelvic floor. Repeat the whole pattern three times, once a day.

A word of comfort: it is almost impossible to do this the first few times. Just get the idea of doing what is asked and persevere. After a few weeks you will achieve control over the different parts of the pelvic floor.

Exercise 5. Now we are going to learn the four different levels of *conscious controlled breathing:* First you learn them simply as a mechanical exercise, and you do them sitting upright—which is fairly easy. Only when the breathing has become more skilful, will you learn to combine this skill with the most important understanding of how and when you will need to use it during labour.

(A) Sit upright on a chair and place the edge of your palm

or tips of fingers in the arch of your rib-cage just above your tummy muscles. In this way you will find the edge of your spread diaphragm. Now, with your mouth closed, take a deep breath, expanding your chest as much as you can. As you do this you will notice the diaphragm going downwards, as it flattens. Now blow the air out through your mouth . . . at the same time note how the muscle rides up again. Repeat this breathing two or three times, keeping the edge of your hand or fingers pressed on the diaphragm.

Ensure that the breathing is gentle and as quiet as possible in each level. The speed should gradually accelerate from Level A to Level C but at a rate and a rhythm which are comfortable for you. Each human being has a slightly different breathing-speed which is comfortable and it is this which is needed for this exercise and later for labour itself. A good test is that your breathing is more visible (the movement of the chest muscles) than audible. (B) Move your hand up to your lower rib-cage, and with your mouth slightly open, breathe in and out, a little less deeply than before. You will notice that your effort now expands the rib-cage under your hand rather than concentrating on your diaphragm.

Make the breath OUT more emphatic than the breath in.

(C) Move your hand up to cover your breastbone. Now breathe still more lightly, so that your main effort is felt in this position.

Think of the word "out" and say it in your mind each time you breath out. Notice that the breath in, follows naturally.

(D) Relax your chest and shoulders completely, so that the ribs are down and the muscles slack. Do not concentrate on your breathing any longer, but let it happen automatically, as it usually does. Instead of thinking of your breathing, choose a song, which you like and of which you know the words. Don't choose a nursery-song because this is too simple. Rather find a pop-song or some other one you are fond of, which also has a good rollicking rhythm. Now sing the song in your head, mime it with your lips, and tap the rhythm with your fingers on the table, or on your lap. Always use the same song when practising and also later during labour—make it *your song*. Particularly, exaggerate the miming with your lips, because this activity of the muscles surrounding the mouth helps a great deal when you are trying to maintain control over your muscles.

Practise this exercise every day using about half a minute for each level. Obviously it's going to help if you can have a clock with a second-hand nearby. Try and learn to make the change smoothly from one level to the next, and change immediately, without having to think. If you or your husband drive a car you will understand easily if I remind you that this is the same kind of skill you needed when you learned to handle the gears. In fact, you can think of levels (A), (B), (C), and (D) as the four gears in your car if you like. It will help you appreciate all the more, how important it is to "change gear" quickly and smoothly.

Exercise 6: This exercise will help the muscles which support your growing bust; it will also teach a special

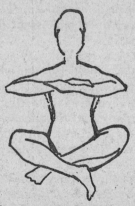

Diagram 8

breathing-drill to be used during the pushing stage of labour.
Sit on the floor "tailor-fashion". Raise your amrs to
shoulder-height. Grip the forearms mutually, above the
wrists. Then push the elbows rhythmically towards each
other: you should feel a definite sensation when you do so,
in the muscles which support your breasts. If you don't feel
anything, raise your arms a little higher.

Combine with breathing as follows: Get arms into
position whilst taking two breaths in and out using Level
(A) breathing. (*) Take a third breath in and *hold it.* Push
your shoulders and ribs downwards and tip your chin on to
your chest. While counting to 10 in your mind, rhythmically push the elbows 10 times towards each other. Release
your breath but keep the arms in position. *Repeat once
from* (*).

Exercise 7. The last exercise for today again has a funny
nickname: the "fallen angel exercise". Its purpose is to
increase the capacity of the upper chest which is used so
much during this conscious controlled breathing.

Sit "tailor-fashion" on the floor. Straighten your shoulders, and hold your arms loosely by your side as though you
were going to use them as wings. Using Level (B) breathing,
lift your arms a little, while breathing in, then let them drop
while breathing out.

Repeat—but lift arms to half way up the body. Then
repeat lifting arms to shoulder-height and dropping them
halfway down the body. Lastly, lift to shoulder-height and
on breathing out, let them drop to the floor. Next repeat the
whole exercise one more BUT this time with your arms still,
palms facing upwards and elbows turned backwards, so that
you feel a pull in your upper arm muscles while doing the
exercise.

Now you will probably collapse wondering if this mass of
things to do is going to grow at this alarming rate! It isn't.
During the coming week you should practise *all* these

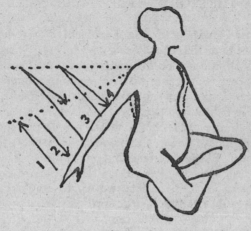

Diagram 9

exercises you have learned in lesson 1 and 2, but after lesson 3 we will start to replace some of the exercises with new ones. So then you won't have too many to practise all together.

THE STORY OF REPRODUCTION

EACH time I give a lecture on the subject of reproduction I
have a faint hope that I shall never have to do so again. Why?
Because it should not be the business of some "authority"
to teach other people about the normal functioning of their
own bodies. From time immemorial, *mothers* have taught
their children how to keep their bodies clean, have taught
them how to use the tools which one uses to put food into
one's mouth, have taught them also the basic skills of social
relationships. But as for teaching one's own children how
mankind procreates! There is a very strong taboo on this!

In modern Western society we try to compromise by
artificial, authoritative instruction on the reproductive
function. A young mother once said at the end of her
"lesson 3": "You know we learnt biology at school, but
somehow it was very difficult to imagine that I and the
bunny-rabbit have that much in common." It should not be
a biology mistress's job to teach young people how their
bodies function any more than it should be mine. So I hope
you will make it your job to teach *your* own children how
their reproductive system works. It shouldn't be a formal
lecture. Not the "Come-along-children-I-have-something-
to-tell-you" approach. But the gradual introduction of
aspects he or she can absorb as they arise naturally in the
course of living; an honest, simple answer to a question
asked by your child whenever some happening stimulates
his thoughts on the subject of his own body.

An anecdote about my own children might amuse you.
(By the way, my children have never had formal teaching
about reproduction but have heard the subject referred to
so often that I have long been confident each knew as much
as he or she could cope with.) My daughter (aged eleven)

and my son (aged eight) were discussing the necessity of being married in order to have a child. I walked in, to find them in a middle of a fine old argument! "Mummy, do explain to him that one must be married to have a baby" pleaded the young woman. I said to my son: "Look, you know very well that a woman can have a baby without her husband being there, but that the baby's father has to put his seed into the mother's body so that the baby can grow in the first place". The young man of eight looked at me as though I needed instruction and said with slow emphasis: "I know that, you silly, but they don't have to be married for that. Haven't you heard of unmarried mothers?"

We then had twenty minutes discussion about the social structure but on the subject of reproduction his views were in no need of clarification. This should be no more a matter for embarrassment than the fact that all human beings put food into their mouths. But in order not to be embarrassed, we must understand the function of reproduction clearly and it must be related to our own bodies. Hence the following lesson. It should be background information for you, so that you can understand the function of labour better; it should also serve as the basis for your own teaching of your children.

In the picture on page 60 you see the contents of the pelvic basin in a fully mature but non-pregnant woman. She is shown lying on her back. The tummy muscles have been cut away, so that you can look at her as it were in cross-section. You can see the coccyx, or tailbones attached at the bottom of the sacrum; then there is a thick layer of muscle with a sort of channel running through it.

That channel is the last part of the large bowel which ends with a tight muscle guarding the exit from the back passage. The correct name for this is the *rectum*. Another bit of muscle wall divides it from the next channel, one with which you are familiar—the vagina. And dipping into the vagina from the top of the pelvic basin is a muscular bag, looking rather like a small, deflated football bladder—the womb, or the word you will hear all the time in pregnancy, the *uterus*. In a non-pregnant woman this is about the size of a pear.

Then comes more muscle wall, and the urinary bladder, with a thin pipe called the *urethra* leading to the outside. Next, more muscle going up to the tummy; then a pad of fat which sits over the junction of the pubic bones, protecting the pubic arch very effectively against injury.

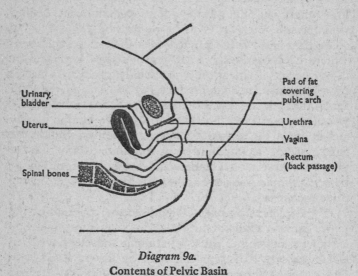

Diagram 9a.
Contents of Pelvic Basin

Now let's look at the next diagram on page 66. You'll see we're now looking at our non-pregnant woman from the front, and the uterus has been deliberately enlarged so you can see it clearly. It has also been cut in half to show the inside rather like an apple cut in half. Do you see the thick muscular wall, roughly triangular in shape, and much narrower at the bottom? The wider bit at the top is called the *body* of the uterus. The narrow bit is called the *cervix* or neck of the womb. In connection with obstetrics, the neck of the womb is almost invariably referred to as the cervix: this is something you must know about, because the cervix undergoes important changes in the course of labour; these are caused by the activity of the body of the uterus. You will notice that the muscular wall encloses a chamber. This is the "nursery" which expands with the growing baby—which is more than you can say for any other nursery your baby might have! Running down through the cervix is a corridor which comes out of the body of the uterus and connects directly with the vagina.

Two extensions from the top of the uterus on either side are two tubes with finger-like endings: these are the *Fallopian tubes*. And they encircle two small, almond-shaped organs, one on either side called the *ovaries*—or if you like, egg-factories, which is what they are.

Whether you are carrying a boy or a girl is something I *can't* tell you. But in either case, if you are over 25 weeks pregnant, your baby is by now completely formed. It has all its organs—lungs, stomach, liver, intestines and its reproductive organs. So if you're carrying a little girl she already has a vagina, uterus, Fallopian tubes, ovaries, but terribly tiny, of course, and not functioning yet.

The reason why I'm telling you this is an interesting one. As the baby is born, your body gives its body a sort of last boost so that all its organs are stimulated and given a really good start to independent life. This includes the reproductive organs, too. So if you have a baby girl, you may notice some time during the first four or five days after she is born, that when you change her nappy, there are a few drops of blood in it.

Now your first thought may be "Ugh . . . blood, haemorrhage, disease!" But she's not ill—she's menstruating! That boost to the reproductive system causes a slight menstrual discharge. It only happens once. And it's not gallons, but literally only two or three drops. If she has had her bowels open in the same nappy you won't know unless you send every nappy to the laboratory. But if you do see this, don't be alarmed, because that's all it is.

Well then, for many years afterwards—anything from twelve to sixteen—nothing more seems to happen. It is just as if the reproductive system apparently didn't function in little girls. But it's not true—it does. From the age of a few weeks, it is growing as the rest of the girl's body is growing; and from the age of about seven or eight it begins to function in various different ways. As it develops towards maturity, all sorts of other changes take place in the body; all sorts of emotional changes occur too, because emotions are related to biological function, although we don't normally *connect* the two.

Let me give you some examples of this connection so that you can recognise them if you see them in your own child. (They occur in little boys too, by the way, but differently— related to becoming a mature male). Here's one thing for instance, that a little girl will do. Say you decide to put her into panties instead of nappies for the first time. She's been pretty dry recently and you think you might risk it. (You're so tired of washing nappies anyway!) So you put her into panties and you don't say anything, just to see how it goes. You'll find that within the hour she'll find some man—it could be her father or an uncle, the milkman or the postman, the first man to come along. And she'll say to him "Look, panties!"

You'll be terribly embarrassed. How can *your* daughter behave like this? But your daughter does behave like this because biologically she is already doing a very feminine thing in drawing attention to her body. And it's her instinct to draw this attention unerringly from a man and not from a woman.

At the age of five she will probably find a boy-friend of

perhaps five-and-a-half. But from her point of view this relationship, you will discover, is partly maternal. She will protect him. She will try to do what she thinks will please him. I remember vividly my son's girl friend when he was six, six-and-a-half, or seven. She used to wander around behind him, all big-eyed; she even went so far as being interested in cars! But unfortunately, he soon reached the age of eight. And at the age of eight little boys are not interested in little girls. Girls are not interested in boys either, for that matter. This is the period when one wants to work in groups of one's own sex.

But of course she hadn't yet reached that stage. I used to see her trotting forlornly about the garden, looking for him. Whenever she saw me she'd say "Where's Nicholas?" "He's out playing." "Oh!" And she would walk away, so sadly—very much the broken-hearted woman. I was so sorry for her that I felt I wanted to produce another son for her, just to keep her going until she got to around eight or nine when it wouldn't matter.

The next period of direct interest in the male develops at around ten and onwards. And it develops into a sort of symbolic interest because the male who interests her from ten onwards is one who is unattainable. This is the secret of the success behind the teenage beat groups and pop stars. In the past, film stars were more in vogue than now for much the same reason. You see, if any one of these girls who swoon and tear the ties off their idols could actually have one of these boys (quite nice boys, really, I'm sure) all to herself, she just wouldn't know what to do with him! This is why it's a good thing that they are protected by their glamour against becoming involved with any of their fans. And all the time this external stimulus is fascinating them, their internal system is constantly growing and preparing for the next stage of their development.

Round about the age of twelve to sixteen, the first human egg begins to develop in a girl's body. Even before she was born, her body contained in each ovary 200,000 yolk specks, which is another way of saying unripe eggs. Yes, 200,000—that means there are 400,000 altogether! Obviously we don't use up 400,000. But nature makes sure that there are plenty. In fact there must be an excess.

The female egg is just like any other egg. It has a yolk, an egg-white, and a shell. Not the hard shell you are accustomed to in the eggs you normally meet, whether they have little lions on or not. Birds' eggs have hard shells because their young develop outside the mother's body, and there isn't much protection outside. So each young bird develops inside its own egg and is protected by this hard shell. Otherwise the species just couldn't survive. But the young human enjoys the luxury of being able to develop inside the mother's body. So the human egg doesn't need a hard shell—just a very fine skin surrounding the "yolk" and the "egg-white". You've met this in the hen's egg too. When you hardboil an egg and peel it, you get that sort of thin white stuff which always seems to end up under your fingernails, and has to be rinsed off. This is the *true* shell of the egg; all eggs have this, as well as the other hard one which you only get if the young develop outside the mother's body.

So, sometimes in a girl's middle teens, the first egg ripens inside her ovaries. And when the egg is fully ripe, still microscopically small but quite complete, the ovary does something with it. It spits it out, so to speak. Soon one of the finger-like ends of the Fallopian tube comes into contact with it. The tube picks up the egg and sucks it inside—it does this partly with its own movement and partly with tiny hairs in its lining, which help to move the egg in the direction in which it is intended to go. So the egg sets off on its journey along the Fallopian tube to the uterus, which may take anything from eight to seventy-two hours.

While this is going on, something else is happening too. The uterus prepares for its reception. But the uterus is only interested in receiving an egg which is fertilized—that is, which potentially can become a baby. So it behaves as though it were fertilized. It begins to store food for the "visitor"—rather like you and I might behave just before Christmas.

Let us say that we have invited three people to lunch on Christmas Day. But we aren't quite sure whether only three people are going to come—or whether half the street is going to take it into its head to come and wish us a Merry Christmas! So we begin to fill our larder several weeks earlier with tins of this and bottles of that. And by Christmas Eve the larder is pretty well near to bursting point.

This is what the uterus does. In blood vessels behind the lining of the womb it begins to store up blood. Now, we tend to think of blood as a nasty red substance which we see if we cut ourselves, and quickly cover up by sticking a bit of plaster on. But blood actually is the carrier of food and oxygen to all the cells in our bodies. Blood ensures that even the tiny cells at the ends of your fingers are well-supplied with food and oxygen. Because if they weren't, they would die. And this little egg is a cell too. So the blood—food in other words—is stored behind the lining of the chamber in the pelvic basin in many tiny blood vessels.

However, when the egg arrives in the uterus nothing happens to it. It just remains an egg. It drops to the bottom of the chamber and there it sits for about 48 hours. Well, there is a limit to how much food you can go on storing when it isn't needed. There's a limit to how much food you can put in *your* larder, too. Beyond a certain point the larder door will come off its hinges! And this happens to the uterus too. About 48 hours after the egg has arrived, the larder door comes off its hinge. The lining breaks up and blood begins to ooze out into the chamber. It doesn't stay there; it runs through the connecting corridor out into the vagina, and away. There are about two to four ounces of blood stored and as you know, it takes several days to get rid

5

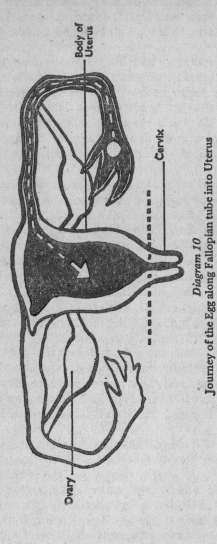

Diagram 10

Journey of the Egg along Fallopian tube into Uterus

of it. And the egg is just washed out along with it.

As soon as all the blood has gone, the lining repairs itself. Then the same process starts all over again. But this time the *other* ovary produces the egg. And it works like that in January, February, June, and July—unless and until one of the ovaries doesn't function for some reason or has to be removed. If this happens then the second ovary takes over the job of both.

Now it takes about thirteen or fourteen days from the beginning of a period for the egg to ripen. The time needed for a fertilized egg to establish itself in the uterus and start using the stored-up blood supply is another ten days or so. When this doesn't happen, during the next few days the extra blood-supply to the uterus is cut off and the unwanted "food" in the lining is disposed of. And since this process repeats itself monthly, so we get the familiar monthly rhythm of round about 26 to 28 days which repeats itself again and again and again. And that is how and why our monthly periods are as they are.

Now let's think about what happens if other factors come in. The ovary has produced an egg and it is already in the Fallopian tube. While this is happening the girl has intercourse. And during intercourse, at the moment of the man's sexual climax, round about the area where the opening of the cervix (or corridor to the uterus) leads into the vagina, millions of male seeds (their correct name is *spermotozoa,* a long word, so "male seeds" will do beautifully) are expelled into the vagina with considerable force.

Male seeds look quite different from the egg—rather like a dressmaker's pin with, instead of a straight bit, a sort of lashing tail. They can move too, and they move at a tremendous rate. In fact their main purpose appears to be movement. So there is a great milling activity among the male seeds inside the passage. But remember that they too are microscopically small—you have to have a fairly strong microscope to see them. Many of them get lost in the nooks and crannies of the vagina, of which there are many. These are simply discharged along with the woman's bodily excretions. But many do find their way up the channel of the cervix, and from here they enter the chamber of the uterus. So there they are. And there are two Fallopian tubes. But there are no signs saying "This way, gentlemen, please". So some go up the empty Fallopian tube, and these are again got rid of with the bodily secretions. But some do find their way into the tube with the egg. That's why there are so many, to allow for this.

The first male seed to get to the egg unites with it and these two tiny cells become one cell. But this contains and keeps all the characteristics of the sperm and the egg. This moment when the two cells fuse and become one, is what is called *conception*. This is the moment at which pregnancy begins.

Now this is an important moment. And you would think, wouldn't you, that there would be something . . . I always feel that there ought to be bells ringing and lights flashing, and the sound of a triumphant fanfare from somewhere. On the contrary, nothing like that happens at all! Can *you* tell when you conceived? You might know when you had intercourse. Perhaps it was Saturday evening: your husband had taken you out to dinner, you both felt good and wanted to make love. But since this moment of conception could have taken place within 60 minutes or 60 hours after that exciting occasion, you don't know when it actually was, I don't know and nobody knows. It takes place silently and secretly.

But it doesn't stay like that. Within a few minutes of conception a cell division takes place and a cluster of cells develops, looking not unlike a bunch of grapes. All these cells contain potentially the physical characteristics not only of mother, owner of the Fallopian tube and the original egg, and of father, original owner of the sperm, but of all their ancestors behind them too.

So if you don't like your baby's flattened toenails or double-jointed thumbs, don't blame your husband! What on earth do you know about the conditions of the toenails of your great-great-great-grandfather? With every baby that is conceived, the particular combination is unique, but the number of combinations of such possibilities is virtually endless, or "infinite", as we say.

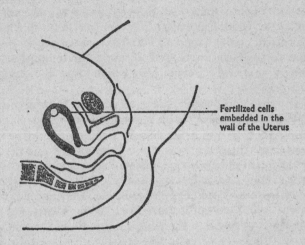

Fertilized cells embedded in the wall of the Uterus

Diagram 11
Pelvic Basin after conception

Well now, the Fallopian tube pushes this cluster of cells towards the uterus—and now all that storing of food and oxygen begins to have some point. When the cluster of cells reaches the uterus it embeds itself in the spongy wall. Immediately, extra blood is diverted to that spot to feed and oxygenate the cluster of cells. Otherwise the cells wouldn't survive. And this time there is no shedding of the lining. Or if there is some excess and a slight break does occur, the amount got rid of is scanty in comparison with the normal amount. This is why the absence of a menstrual period, or at least a very scanty one as opposed to one's usual one, is usually the first indication a woman has that she might be pregnant.

At this point, all sorts of fascinating changes take place. But you don't know about them because you can't feel them. It would be wonderful if we could see or feel them, or experience them in some way. But all anyone can do is to describe them. And you ought to know, at least in retrospect, what happened! The next diagram illustrates very roughly what happens. The first menstrual period that ought to be, hasn't appeared. If you could look inside the uterus you would see something which looks like this spot in diagram 11.

I suppose you'll agree that even with the best intentions in the world, it doesn't look much like your dream child. It doesn't look like your husband's family, either. But two weeks later—in other words you have missed one period, you are a fortnight overdue and you are beginning to think as one usually does in terms of baby clothes—something else interesting has already happened inside. The cluster of cells has divided. Two-thirds have sort of separated and are beginning to grow into the *embryo*—the tiny form that will later be the body of your son or daughter. One-third has remained attached, usually in the top part of the uterus. This is developing into a special organ which will act as a filter for food and oxygen taken from your circulation and used to supply your baby.

It also acts as a filter in the opposite direction. As the little embryo grows, growth produces waste. And waste has to be got rid of. The only way you can do this is through the mother's own blood-supply, out through her kidneys, her skin and her bowels. A rope of blood vessels attaches the embryo to this organ.

The name of this organ is the *placenta,* or the word you

will hear much more often, the *after-birth*. Although the placenta is so vitally necessary to the developing baby until it is born, after it is born it can breathe and eat and so fend for itself in terms of food and oxygen. Then the placenta is no longer needed, and will be "born" after the baby—hence the name of after-birth.

Some midwives have another name for it. After the birth you may be holding your baby in your arms and notice the midwife still apparently fiddling about. And you will say: "Haven't you finished?" If she replies "No, dear, we're waiting for the baby's luggage" then you'll know what she means!

Now, this cord of blood vessels is attached to the baby, right in the middle of its abdomen, or where its abdomen will one day be. It is rather like a climber tied by nylon rope to a piece of rock. Over the placenta there grows a bag rather like a polythene bag, and the baby lives inside it. In fact it floats inside this bag of water. The placenta secretes water and this acts as a buffer. You may have heard of cars which have fluid suspension. But even travelling in a car with fluid suspension is like riding in an old-fashioned horse-and-cart in comparison with the fluid suspension in the uterus around the baby. That's how efficient it is.

Now if we could see it after six weeks we would see something like diagram 12. Now, it's beginning to look recognisable—if you use your imagination! Its head is a little out of proportion but what will one day emerge is beginning to develop. The spinal bones are suspiciously long and there is a kind of vestige of a tail. The arm and leg buds are beginning to be noticeable, too.

A week later the separation from the placenta is much more clear and so is the cord. So at two and a half months' pregnancy—and that means two periods missed plus a fortnight—it's a rather nice but small human being.

There are still things which need improving, of course But at three-and-a-half months' pregnancy, fingernails and

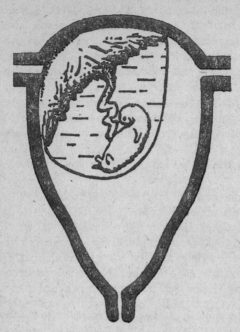

Diagram 12
Six weeks after conception

toenails are visible and sexual organs can be clearly seen. At
four and a half months it is neatly packed into the pelvic
basin And it can do something which neither you nor I can
do, pregnant or otherwise. It can lie there comfortably
tucked up, with its toes tickling its forehead. When you are
no longer pregnant, you try to lie with your toes tickling
your forehead and see how far you get! Still, this is a very
efficient way of packing it so that it is comfortably enclosed
and has room to move its body. The placenta and the cord
can be clearly seen.

By seven months the embryo is rather handsome. The

placenta is firmly attached to the umbilical cord. It is upside down, in other words with its head in the pelvic basin. At seven months the baby usually turns and lies like this. Actually it can turn at any old time—sometimes they do it at six months, sometimes not until nine. But seven months is considered to be the moment of perfection. It turns this way of course, because if you are going to wend your way out of a fairly tight channel, if you have any sense you go head first, and not feet first. And this is why 96 out of 100 babies are born this way.

The contents of the pelvic basin at full term look very different from the pelvic basin in a non-pregnant woman. The uterus is expanded just like a football, with the baby floating inside the bag (called, by the way, the *bag of membranes*) attached to the placenta. In fact the uterus is now so large that only part of it can be contained by the pelvis; there are other changes in the pelvic area too, such as the softening of the cervix, the vagina and the joints between the bones, all of which help it to stretch. Everything else is still there—but in the area that once accommodated comfortably a whole lot of organs, among others the uterus, baby's head is now the major occupant. The bladder is still there too, because we can hardly remove it, but only just! Because it gets so squashed, you'll find that towards the end of the pregnancy (much more than now or at the beginning) you'll spend more time in the lavatory than anywhere else.

That is basically the story of the development of pregnancy. Now if the pelvic basin itself has to change this much, and make this much adjustment in accommodation, imagine what happens to the rest of the body. It has to adjust itself not just to nourishing for two, but to things like excreting for two as well. But curiously enough, the food your body supplies to the baby is not the food you eat. The roast chicken and brussels sprouts you eat now are not supplied directly to the baby; they are converted by your

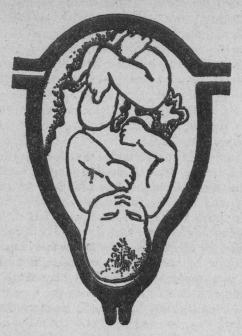

Diagram 13
End of pregnancy (frontal view)

body into reserve supplies which can be sent via your
bloodstream to the baby whenever he needs them. This is
why taking all those vitamin tablets and iron tablets and
things is not so directly important for the baby as it is for
you. So why all this protective feeding? The answer is, it's
for *your* benefit. The Minister of Health wants you to stay
looking beautiful, with glossy hair, all (or most) of your
teeth and a nice skin. This is what it's for and not for just
baby. So if you value *you* as much as you value your baby,
you will take just as much care of yourself.

Any questions? These are some I have been asked:

Q.   When did you say the baby was fully formed?

A.   At 25 weeks roughly.

Q.   Why can't it be born then?

A.   Being fully formed doesn't mean fully functioning. It has to grow in size, and organs have to develop sufficiently to be capable of functioning. At 25 weeks they couldn't. There are another fifteen weeks beyond that, and fifteen weeks is only just under four months. I know pregnancy seems like three years—I have felt by eight months that I've been pregnant all my life. But it isn't really so long, you know. Forty weeks. Less than a year to develop a complete functioning human being from two tiny microscopic cells.

Q.   You said that the coming-out position is usually head down. Can there be any other position? I don't mean in labour, but before that.

A.   Almost any position—lying across for instance, or sitting with the bottom in the pelvic basin. By the way, this is known as the position of *breech*. This is because the part which would present itself first would be covered in breeches as soon as it emerged! ("Breeches" is the old-fashioned word for trousers.)

You will find that the baby will change its position all the time. All the movements a baby makes right from the beginning are muscle development movements. As you have learned, if you don't move your muscles they become very flabby, and you can't use them properly. You know how your legs feel when you've been in bed for a week with 'flu? All jelly-like. Well, although you will discover when your baby is born that its body feels all jelly-like in comparison with your own, if fact, if it hadn't made all the movements it did, this would be even more so. And so you might like to know when you feel those vicious thumps that the baby is doing its exercises!

Later on, when the baby goes right down with its head first, you'll get another sensation which you will definitely *not* like. This is when the baby is strengthening its neck muscles by moving its head against your bladder. It feels rather like being butted by a goat! But when you hold the baby up at six weeks and say proudly, "Look how beautifully he holds his head!" you will have forgotten by then how sore it made you feel.

Perhaps it will comfort you a little if I say that these movements are purposeful and not random. That sort of churning feeling, like someone turning over and over in bed—that's just what it is. And when it feels as though the baby were doing a somersault—it is. Until the baby gets too big, it usually spends its time sitting one way for half-an-hour then moving to another position for another half-hour, then sometimes it doesn't move at all for a bit. It sleeps and wakes just like anyone else.

Q.   It doesn't breathe through its *lungs* in there, does it?

A.   No, it doesn't breathe at all in that sense. But it gets fresh air from the mother's bloodstream via the placenta and the umbilical cord and it gets rid of air the same way.

Q.   How is it known about the baby sleeping and waking?

A.   Some of this information is obtained, watching organisms which are much simpler than the human and making comparisons. But there have been new exciting developments in photography too—and fascinating pictures are emerging from the laboratories which show that the baby's muscles go completely limp like anyone else's when it's curled up in sleep. These were taken in periods when the mothers reported no movements, as though it were asleep! So they were right.

There's a wonderful book, if you're really interested, called "The First Nine Months of Life" which shows a lot of these photographs. I'm sure your library would get it for you.

THE SECRET WEAPON FOR LABOUR:
NEURO-MUSCULAR CONTROL

You cannot help but have heard, unless you have lived in an age of isolation, all your life, of relaxation classes in preparation for childbirth. And you must have heard of people who said, "Well I went to classes and I wouldn't say that they helped me much when the pains got really strong." You may then have wondered why so many of your friends who had been to relaxation classes in preparation for childbirth had such comparatively indifferent results from all the relaxing they did.

I am aware that there are about 12% of women to whom relaxation has been of great value. But there are specific reasons for this. Anyway, 12% of women isn't very many; and you may bet your bottom dollar that you are probably not one of the 12% either. So it doesn't help you much, does it?

To begin with, what fool first dragged up this idea that relaxation classes for childbirth would be the thing? And secondly, why don't I just teach relaxation in my classes? There are very good reasons.

Let's look at the history of this sort of approach. Before the days of Queen Victoria, the idea of passivity during labour was completely unknown. Women did the best they could. They were anything but relaxed and passive; in fact they were often wildly active and uncontrolled. They were also in considerable pain. A famous doctor called Simpson first used chloroform during the birth of one of Queen Victoria's children. This is in fact the first known case in history—although there were legendary cases before it—of a woman being rendered passive with benefit during the birth of her child. It was the administration of chloroform that made her passive; you can give anyone chloroform and they'll become passive. I once worked in a laboratory where there was a bottle of chloroform which was used for all sorts of things. One day our cleaner was dusting the shelves and dropped the bottle of chloroform. She became passive too . . .

After Simpson, it was soon discovered that giving chloroform could be slightly risky both for mother and child. For although it rendered them passive it also rendered their involuntary activities like breathing, somewhat passive too. And the mother would actually breathe hardly at all. So the baby's respiratory follow-up or in other words, the oxygen the baby should get from the placenta and which was not being supplied, wasn't much either. And everybody had a fairly unhappy time.

From Queen Victoria's time until the 1940's constant efforts were being made by research workers in the medical profession to produce better and safer drugs that would render women passive in labour more safely. And it was gradually realised that if you don't interfere with the working of the uterus in labour by taking energy away from it to use on other muscles and thus waste oxygen, then you were likely to do better.

It was Dr. Dick Read who first said: "Well, yes, passivity is obviously desirable. But why does it have to be induced chemically, with drugs? You can produce it by teaching people to relax. And by teaching mothers the value of not wasting energy and oxygen, and not interfering inadvertently with the activities of the uterus."

Excellent, except for the fact that you can't do it. The theory is sound enough: the more conservation of energy you can create in the course of labour and the more correct the oxygen supply in the course of labour, the more efficiently the uterus will function and the less uncomfortable the woman will feel. And the more happy she will feel. This is the origin of relaxation classes.

But as I said, relaxation doesn't really work except for 12% of women. The reason why is quite simple, but needs some explaining. When we were formed and this goes for all of us—our muscles brought, as it were, very few skills with them. Of course every new-born baby has certain skills, all connected with particular kinds of muscles working in association together. All of these are for the purpose of survival in one way or another. The most obvious one of these you will discover as soon as you meet your baby. Put your finger in his palm; immediately his fingers will grasp yours firmly. Nobody taught him to do this. It is a very good skill to have, particularly if you evolved originally from a species which had to hang on to things in order not to fall off! It's purely biological.

Another muscular skill a new-born baby has is the ability to suck and swallow. Some time you should try taking a bottle, a squash-bottle will do, putting some water or milk or orange juice in it, and sucking and swallowing liquid out of it. Do it very slowly so that you get some idea of how many of your muscles actually have to go into action to perform this. It is so difficult that we tend to give up the practice as we grow up!

When children are four and five they do still like to drink from bottles, because it makes a nice noise. But after this they happily go to a straw: it's even more fun, and it's so much easier. Finally they take to a cup because it's actually less tiring.

Sucking your food in the way a baby does uses an awful lot of muscular energy. Whether it sucks it from a teat or from a breast makes very little difference; in each case, several different groups of muscles work together to produce the ability to suck.

All subsequent activities which we learn, all of us, in the course of growing up, are combinations of muscles working together. The significant thing about all of them is this;

when we first learn them (because we want to do something or other) we find that combining the different groups of muscles which work together is very difficult. Watch a baby at seven or eight months when he is learning to crawl. First he gets the idea that he doesn't want to sit here any more. He wants to go over there—there's something over there he wants to investigate. A nice, bright something. He looks at it over there, and you can see him measuring the distance. Then he will find some way of reaching it. One of the most obvious ways is to buckle your foot underneath your bottom and to do what we call the "Russian hop". This is very fast in the young baby. (It tends to get slower as we get older!)

The other method, of course, is crawling. You'll be surprised if you've never watched anybody crawl, at just how much you have to know, to do it. Which foot should you put first? The back one? Oops—no, that won't help. Try the other one—that's better. Now a bit further . . . soon it becomes an automatic skill until finally the baby is crawling faster than mother can walk, which is all part of the fun. But you will admit that working the muscles in association in order to crawl is a considerable skill. Even if you *do* tend to look down on it once you can walk: no child of eighteen months who can walk would be seen dead, crawling!

All the things which you do later—running, skipping, jumping, climbing—are all done by groups of muscles working together. And when any muscles work, they do so because of a message sent by your brain and prompted by your will: You know—"I want to get over there!" The brain sends the message to the muscles concerned via the nerves: so this is called a *neuro-muscular skill* . . . The simple ability to reach out and grab something, which you acquire at about five months, is a complex neuro-muscular skill. So is the ability to speak; not the formation of words, but the ability to actually use your voice box. Running, jumping, climbing—these are all equally neuro-muscular skills.

Later we have the fascinating business of learning to write. When you write busily away at a letter, you are thinking about what you are writing. You may of course be inventing your own shorthand—but I don't suppose you are thinking about how to hold your pencil. But you did, once. Don't you remember the first time you were given a pencil and tried to write? And how fascinated you were at first by the fact that you could manage to make scribbles all over the paper? Finally it became much more fascinating to do something *deliberate* all over the paper. Then came strokes and then letters. Finally you experienced the joy of mastering a new neuro-muscular skill; you could put together the letters you wanted, to form your name.

The first time you wrote your own name was a real milestone in neuro-muscular development. All of them are acquired in this almost painful way. Yet they become terribly mechanical, just like "changing-gear" breathing is now. When you write now, you don't even think about it any more. You just scribble. You might, if you're signing a cheque, think briefly about the bank manager's possible reaction to this dastardly act. But you don't think any more about how you hold the pen, do you? And if you scrawled your name much faster than you wrote out the amount of the cheque, the reasons have nothing whatever to do with your neuro-muscular skill!

By the time we are fifteen to eighteen years old, we have all acquired thousands of these semi-automatic patterns of neuro-muscular activity, because otherwise life as an adult human being, in the very complex environment we live in would be impossible. Even extra skills like typing, driving a car, playing the piano, using a knitting machine, or just learning ordinary knitting become semi-automatic. These are not just survival skills; they are fun, leisure, creative skills. But all of them are of neuro-muscular origin. So by the time you reach your late teens you have acquired most

6

of yours. We do learn a few more later but by comparison these are very few.

There is no harm in the fact that these skills become mechanical. It is perfectly alright for all ordinary purposes. But it does mean that the brain acquired habits in the way it works. The brain is just a mechanical machine that does the work which we have taught it to do. We therefore have muscles with a strong habit of working together, regardless of whether or not they are needed for a particular activity.

Let me give you an example or two. Supposing you are carrying a heavy shopping-bag. You are using the muscles of one hand and arm—otherwise the bag will drop. The other hand and arm are by no means inactive, by no means at rest. They will try to join in—to mimic what the hand which is in action does. This happens when undertaking any kind of activity connected with a group of muscles ... It doesn't merely work on one's own, neuro-muscular activity either. It works with other people's too. Recently I was watching an opera-singer on television; she was performing the part of a tragic heroine. And I noticed that as she charged about the screen, singing away—*my* muscles were contracted. Because I am so aware of muscles, I was able to decontract as soon as I realised this. But as I watched her fall to her knees, leap to her feet and then stride about again, once again *my* muscles contracted too.

Another interesting thing is what happens when you are walking in very high-heeled shoes. Your feet begin to feel uncomfortable. What do you do? Well, the only thing to do if you can't take your shoes off and walk in bare feet, is to contract the muscles of your foot away from your shoe. That's better—except that as you do this the muscles of your face contract too. If you don't believe this, have a good look at the faces of women shopping or dancing in high-heeled shoes. Don't their faces look tense?

Perhaps now you will begin to understand why relaxation during the whole course of childbirth doesn't work. It's fine, as all muscles are in a relaxed condition, because the very act of decontracting the muscles, obviously produces a condition which *can* be labelled "Relaxation". It's fine in a relaxation class during pregnancy where nothing is contracted, because all the muscles are doing the same thing. And once someone has learned the method of decontracting them, this isn't difficult for any woman to practise at home. The brain associates the action of all muscles whether in a state of contraction or decontraction, so this is something anyone can master.

But in labour the situation is very different. In labour you have one group of muscles contracting as it wants to, to a particular pattern of its own. And when these muscles begin to contract strongly, then other muscles, quite unconnected with this function, do so too: the muscles of the arms, the legs, the back, even the muscles of the face, all try to join in. And this is the typical picture painted so luridly by Victorian fiction writers when they described their women in childbirth. "A terrible groan escaped from her pale lips. Then her hands clutched the bedpost as her whole body was contorted by unendurable agony"—something like that. But all they are *really* describing is neuro-muscular association. Even so, it is rather an uncomfortable endeavour because it consumes so much energy and oxygen. And it's hardly a picture of relaxation, is it?

So what are we going to do? We can't leave you to have a painful labour lasting four or five days. Instead we teach your brain a new neuro-muscular skill—the skill of deliberately keeping apart, muscular activity. This is called NEURO-MUSCULAR DISASSOCIATION. This is a basically simple, almost mechanical skill, just like walking, for instance, and the application of this skill to labour is relatively easy. Relatively compared to relaxation classes, that is.

Now by this page of the book you should have already
learned a number of completely new physical skills—which
by now are semi-automatic. You should, for instance, be
able fairly easily to "change gear" as part of conscious
controlled breathing. You should be able to combine this
breathing—or at least Level "A" breathing—with controlled
muscular exercise almost as a matter of course, as for
example, in limbering up. So now you should be able to
learn how to use this new "secret weapon", and discover
why it is such an important one for the preparation of an
expectant mother.

The idea that relaxation is of value during childbirth is
now no longer new or inflammatory. But *why* is it
desirable? Well you will remember from Lesson 1 that
muscles use extra oxygen when they are working. And they
also use extra body-energy, more than what is needed
during an ordinary day's work for anyone. This is why men
who are engaged in heavy manual labour need more food;
they have also learned how to combine their work with
deeper breathing, almost without thinking about it. In one
sense giving birth to a child is heavy physical work
too—hence "labour"!

During this event, the group of muscles called the
UTERUS works very hard over several hours to deliver the
baby from the mother's body into the outside world. So
although it isn't manual labour, the muscles are still working
far more than usual. And *as we cannot tell the uterus to rest
when we choose to, we must prepare for constant work*.
This is why it is important for all other physical activity to
be reduced as much as possible, and so make the maximum
body energy and oxygen available for the uterine muscles to
use: if other muscles also go into action when the uterus
does, they are wasting energy and oxygen which should be
in reserve for the uterus. Then the body generally will tire
quickly and prevent the uterus from functioning as efficiently as it should. This is why it is hardly surprising if the

poor Victorian heroines were apparently in labour for days and days! The writers were quite correct: Such behaviour would make the uterus work so inefficiently that delivering the baby might well take that long. (I often wonder how the novelists knew this.)

Fortunately it is only necessary to teach this new exercise to our brain in principle, after which it becomes possible to make the correct use of this principle during labour. We need not use the muscles of the uterus to practise it, but we can use any muscles we like. So for practical purpose we use our arm and leg muscles, as you will see from the diagrams, and "pretend" while the brain is learning this new skill, that our arm and leg muscles are the uterus. And we combine the learning of this neuro-muscular skill with conscious controlled breathing. For this exercise you should lie down in the basic position.

DISASSOCIATION DRILL

The purpose of this drill is to approximate having a uterine contraction during the first stage of labour. You are maintaining all muscles in a state of decontraction, whilst a specific muscle group is contracted.

Contract Left arm: Maintain this for half a minute whilst using Level "A" breathing and maintaining decontraction of all other muscles.

Contract R. arm and R. leg: Repeat drill as before
Contract L. arm and R. leg: ,,   ,,   ,,
Contract R. arm and L. leg: ,,   ,,   ,,

Gradually lengthen the time for each phase of the drill over a period of days as your ability to maintain the state of disassociation increases: when you have lengthened each phase to approximately 45 seconds combine it with the following variations:

While doing the third and fourth phase of Disassociation Drill, ask your husband or a friend to give you the commands for the variations:

When you begin to contract one arm and the opposite leg take:

3 breaths in Level A, then

4-6 breaths in Level B, then

8-10 breaths in Level C, then

15-20 seconds of Level D—in other words, for 15-20 seconds you sing your tune in your head and drum its rhythm with your fingers whilst allowing your chest to breathe naturally.

Then come down through C, B and A again, maintaining your contractions all the time and checking that no other muscles have joined in against your wish. If they have, just correct this but carry on the deliberate contraction *at the same time.*

It is very much easier to develop this skill if someone does your daily practice of this disassociation-drill with you. The other person tells you when to begin, and when to finish each phase, using a watch to time you. Then on the "variation" he or she counts your breaths and varies the numbers as indicated. This is so that you become accustomed to responding instantly to signals which are outside your own conscious control. In labour the signals from the uterus are also outside your conscious control and you should have plenty of practice before labour in making such responses.

Now we discontinue the following exercises: (1) active decontraction-drill, and (2) the separate exercise of the four levels of conscious controlled breathing, once you have started on the "variation".

Both these are of course contained in the disassociation-drill.

Practise this exercise for about ten days and then begin work on Lesson 4.

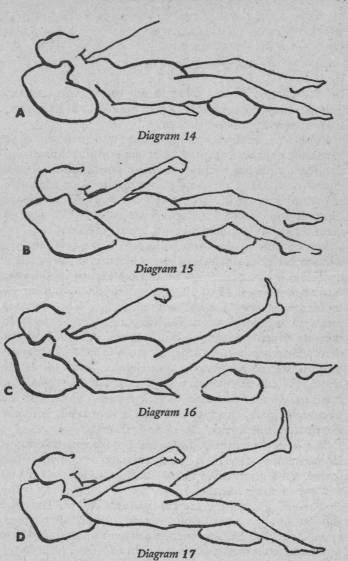

Diagram 14

Diagram 15

Diagram 16

Diagram 17

Lesson 4

B-DAY!

IN this chapter we are going to put together for the first time all that we have learned up to now—and in its correct context in relationship to labour.

But before we discuss what *we* have to do in labour, let's have a look for a moment at what the uterus is expected to do. The uterus has a unique problem during labour. It is a purely mechanical problem but it results in considerable effort on the part of the uterus. Now you will experience this and you should be able to contribute to it in order to make those efforts valuable and the result efficient.

Look at the diagrams on page 228. In the first one you will see the pregnant woman with her uterus fully expanded. The pregnancy is just before the end of its term; in other words this is 39 to 40 weeks after conception and 40 to 41 weeks after the last normal period. The uterus is prepared to go into action. The baby is fully grown ready to take up independent life. You can see the body of the uterus, hugely expanded to accommodate baby plus placenta, plus bag of membranes, plus liquid. There too is the cervix, the corridor between the uterus and the vagina or as it is now correct to call it, the birth canal; along this the baby will finally pass into the outside world. But before it can do that, this corridor has to be dealt with.

You will always hear doctors and midwives talk about labour in *three* stages. (The peculiar jargon of midwifery can sound quite frightening but when you understand it you will see why it is like that.) They will say: "She's still in the first stage". "Hurry up, she's second staging" or "Only the third stage to go now!" And you might think "Oh heavens, what on earth's happening?" unless you understand these terms and what they mean in the right context.

To begin at the beginning: What happens in the first stage of labour? To understand this better we have shown the uterus in Diagram 18, see page 92, from the front, and without the top as it is not necessary. The baby is sitting inside. The corridor (cervix) and vagina (birth-canal) are both indicated. Running through the corridor as you can see is a sort of small passage, in reality very narrow, along which in a non-pregnant woman, the menstrual flow would pass out into the vagina, and the male sperm would pass up into the uterus, and from there into the Fallopian tube for conception to take place.

But now we don't want conception to take place, we want a baby to be born. You can see the baby's head would fill the lower area pretty fully with the cervix acting as a barrier between uterus and birth-canal. And this is when the plain question "How do you get out of here?" must be answered. If you turn the book upside down a minute and look again at diagram 18, perhaps it may remind you of something. A fat bottle, perhaps with a thin neck? It always makes me think of the green wine bottles which tourists buy to bring back for their friends ... you know, instead of "Present from Blackpool" this is a "Present from Athens". Usually the wine is very inferior wine and it is more fun to stand the bottle on one's mantelpiece. However, if you feel like sampling the contents this isn't difficult—these bottles are usually made of clay so you just knock the top off and pour. Then you throw the little bottle away, hoping that your friends will go to Athens again next year and bring you another one. But we can't do that. You can't go back to wherever the uterus came from and buy another one because this isn't clay, this is muscle—living muscle. So what do you do?

Well, *you* don't do anything. But the body of the uterus does. First of all, it pulls the cervix up towards itself thus making it shorter and/or thinner. (Both expressions are used: the shortening of the cervix or the thinning of the cervix. It all depends on your viewpoint!) This goes on until the thickness of the cervix is not greater than the thickness of the wall of the uterus itself. But the opening is still much too small to allow a nice solid baby of anything from seven to ten pounds to come out. It just won't come out, not even mechanically. So the body of the uterus then performs its second job during the first stage of labour; it pulls up the cervix all round so that the opening enlarges rather like the diaphragm of the camera being opened. For all apparent practical purposes no cervix remains; both the body of the uterus and the birth canal become one continuous structure. Next the baby's head slips from the uterus into the birth canal—and then the *second stage of labour,* usually called the expulsive stage, begins. In other words this is the stage during which the body of the uterus (again it is always the body of the uterus which is in action) pushes the baby along the birth canal and out. Your tummy muscles assist in this process, but that is secondary.

So the first stage of labour in fact consists of two stages. The first one we don't even count in fact as a true labour phase. The thinning or shortening of the cervix is a pre-labour phase, followed by the true *first stage of labour,* that of pulling the cervix open. This is called the phase of *dilatation.* (We use the Latin term—it means "opening".) And again you will hear the midwives' jargon: "She is dilating nicely!" If you didn't know you might wonder "Where am I dilating nicely?" There are, of course all sorts of openings where you could be dilating. Well, now you know which one they mean.

From outside, the size of the opening is measured by the midwife's or doctor's fingers. But by you it is measured with a completely different yardstick which you'll learn about shortly. But a midwife or doctor can only go by measurement with fingers. The midwife obviously can't see it because she can't look inside there but she can feel it with two fingers, during an internal examination. She may say

"Hum! She's not dilating yet, she's not really in labour".

But two or three hours later she comes along with her two fingers and this time she might say "Good Heavens! I can put two fingers in and there is more room. Now there's another finger's worth of room. This woman is three fingers dilated." A little later she says: "Look—my two fingers could do a journey in there! She is four fingers, because now four fingers would fit in there. Next, all the cervix at the back will be taken up but around the sides and in front there will be a little left; this is three-quarters dilatation."

And finally she comes in, and there is no cervix. All she meets all round is the baby's head, because as the cervix opens, baby's head comes down lower and lower and lower. In fact what she can feel with her fingers all the time is baby's head or part of baby's head, enough to cover two fingers, then two fingers and a bit, then three, then four fingers until you get full dilatation.

How does the body of the uterus do this? In the same way in which any muscle does anything. Muscle only works by contraction. And the body of the uterus is a group of muscles. So, this process of thinning or shortening followed by dilatation is accomplished by a series of progressive contractions, progressive in the sense that in order to thin the cervix the uterus does not at first have to work very hard. Contractions can be weak and short. But as it gets closer and closer to full dilatation, it has to work much harder, each bit requiring greater effort. So the contractions become longer and much stronger. And the different sensations you feel when the uterus contracts will be your "yardstick" to tell you what to do.

That, in essence, is how the uterus solves its problem of getting the baby into the birth canal. This does not yet explain what you do. Perhaps it would be nice if you could take your uterus to the hospital and leave it there when it is ready to go into action. Then you could go out and enjoy yourself while it gets on with the job collect it again on

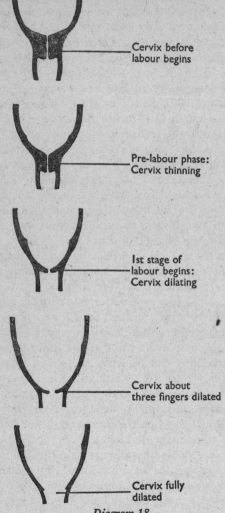

Cervix before
labour begins

Pre-labour phase:
Cervix thinning

1st stage of
labour begins:
Cervix dilating

Cervix about
three fingers dilated

Cervix fully
dilated

Diagram 18
How the Cervix changes during the first stage of
labour

completion—and your baby as well. However, this is just a wistful joke. Whether we like it or not, you and the uterus are linked together and you are going to be there while it does its work. And since you are there you might just as well be useful. All the things we shall learn are aimed at making you capable of doing just that—being useful and enhancing the efficient functioning of your own body-mechanism and at the same time creating maximum comfort for yourself.

Now, even if you were unconscious, vast quantities of both energy and oxygen would be used to perform this pattern of progressive contracting over a period of time. So much so that when dilatation begins, all processes which are not so to speak entirely necessary to survival are quite naturally cut down. The process of digestion is one of them.

Digestion is reduced to a minimum during labour and this gives us some clue as to whether you can eat or not. Circulation of blood to those tissues which can survive for the time being on a smaller supply, is also diminished. And so a woman in labour might be boiling hot up above from all the activity but her feet will be freezing. And she won't just have cold feet because she is naturally one of these people who have cold feet, even women who usually have warm feet have cold feet in labour. And so that you don't have that additional worry "Oh my God, as if all this weren't enough, now I've got cold feet", we always suggest that you put socks on, simply for your comfort. This is because the body itself tries to conserve energy for the uterus to use and tries to save oxygen from functions which it could well do some other time, not now.

And here is where your job comes in. Because you yourself do the job of conserving energy by the process of neuro-muscular disassociation; the constant establishment of disassociation of all muscles not involved with uterine function in labour (See Lesson 3). In other words, your constant job is to keep all other muscles completely decontracted so that they don't waste energy.

You also have to maintain the correct extra supply of oxygen as the body demands it during labour. But you mustn't think that this is like cough mixture—you know, if one tablespoonful of it does you good then three table-spoonfuls ought by simple arithmetic to do three times as much good. It isn't true, actually, either for cough mixture or for labour! It isn't supplying vast amounts of oxygen that matters but *supplying the correct amount at the correct time.* One thing I cannot emphasise too much: the success of what you are trying to do depends upon your disciplined actions and not on the behaviour of your uterus alone. Your mental determination to try your best throughout labour to use your tools exactly will determine how well controlled you remain; your husband's role during labour will be mainly one of strengthening this determination. And he can give you valuable help in using the tools which you will be taught to use. But before you can use your determination in this way, you must know what tools to use—and when.

The *Labour Diagrams* which follow this and the next three lessons are your aid. Look at Labour Diagram (1) on pages 96 and 97. The thick lines represent the actions of the uterus. The zig-zag lines represent the kind of conscious controlled breathing needed for each phase of labour. You will notice that in Labour Diagram (1) the curves are short, and do not rise very much from the straight line. This is a visual representation of the sort of gentle uterine contraction you will experience during the *pre-labour* phase. As these contractions are so gentle, your tummy-muscles will hardly be involved with the action of the uterus, and thus you can breathe comfortably in Level A throughout the whole contraction. If you turn to pages 98, 99, and look at Labour Diagram (2) you will see that the curve looks much more as though it meant business. This diagram represents the kind of contraction you will feel when labour is establishing—in other words, at the beginning of the *phase of dilatation.* Here, although the contractions begin as gently as before, they become stronger after a few seconds and then even stronger. With the increasing strength of uterine action more and more of your tummy-muscles will be involved and thus your controlled breathing must change or you will be uncomfortable.

So, with the increasing strength of sensation during the contractions, you change up from *Level A* through *Level B* into *Level C* breathing, which is usually perfectly adequate for comfort at this stage of labour. After a little while of breathing in *Level C* you will notice that you feel the contraction weakening again. So you come down into *Level B* and finally as it wanes, again into *Level A*. So you make up the oxygen as and when you can. Turn over to Labour Diagram (3), pages 100, 101 and your heart may well miss a beat. Even in diagrammatic terms, progress has obviously been considerable. Indeed, Labour Diagram (3) looks as though life were one long contraction! Many women have said that it felt like that, too, during labour. The contractions are much longer lasting, and become very strong, much faster. This considerably shortens the intervals between them too.

However, your handling remains similar. At the height of this kind of contraction, which you will generally not experience until after three fingers' dilatation of the cervix, you need *Level D* breathing. (The light natural breathing which your chest will automatically adopt if you concentrate *hard* on your tune and beating its rhythm with your fingers.) As the contraction fades again, you come down through the levels with it, making up the oxygen debt created by the vigorous activity of the uterus. When you feel that the contraction has gone, take an extra breath in *Level A* to ensure that your tummy-muscles are at rest. After that, you can wipe your brow, sip some water and discuss the Italian Renaissance if you want to. The trade union rules for women in labour say that when the uterus is not working you don't work either!

LABOUR DIAGRAM I

PRE-LABOUR PHASE-The cervix is thinning; Level A breathing.
Mock contraction for practice: use one arm and same leg.

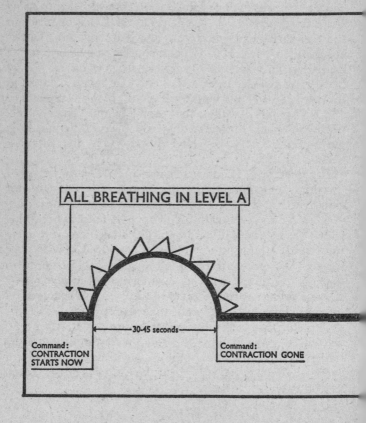

ALL BREATHING IN LEVEL A

—30-45 seconds—

Command:
CONTRACTION
STARTS NOW

Command:
CONTRACTION GONE

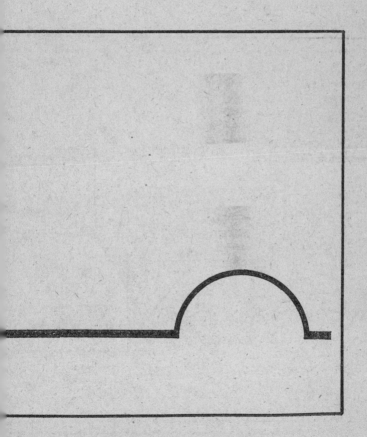

LABOUR DIAGRAM 2

FIRST STAGE OF LABOUR: I—Cervix begins to dilate; change
breathing levels during each contraction. Mock contraction for
practice: one arm and opposite leg (cross-contraction).

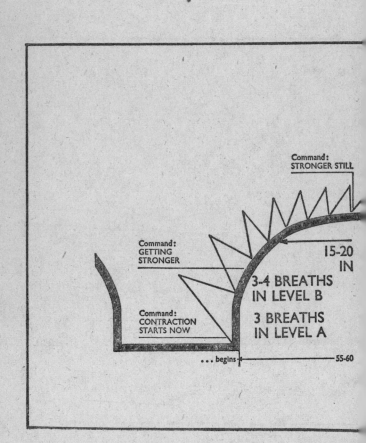

Command:
STRONGER STILL

Command:
GETTING
STRONGER

Command:
CONTRACTION
STARTS NOW

15-20
IN

3-4 BREATHS
IN LEVEL B

3 BREATHS
IN LEVEL A

... begins

55-60

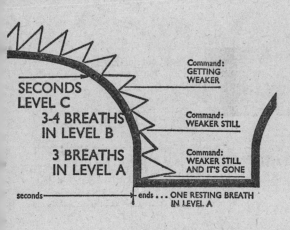

SECONDS
LEVEL C

3-4 BREATHS
IN LEVEL B

3 BREATHS
IN LEVEL A

seconds —————————→ ends ... ONE RESTING BREATH
IN LEVEL A

Command:
GETTING
WEAKER

Command:
WEAKER STILL

Command:
WEAKER STILL
AND IT'S GONE

LABOUR DIAGRAM 3

FIRST STAGE OF LABOUR: II—Dilatation continues; contractions becoming longer and much stronger. Change breathing levels to include Level D. Mock contraction for practice: use opposite arm and leg to Labour Diagram 2 (opposite cross-contraction).
Note: alternative pattern is shown on outer curve.

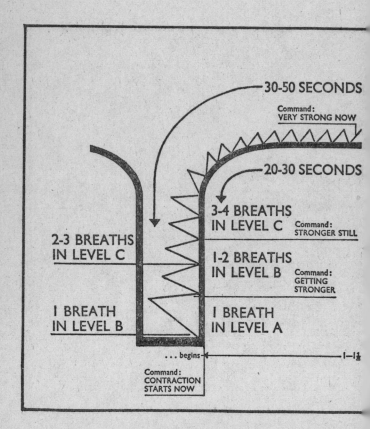

30-50 SECONDS

Command:
VERY STRONG NOW

20-30 SECONDS

3-4 BREATHS
IN LEVEL C
Command:
STRONGER STILL

2-3 BREATHS
IN LEVEL C

1-2 BREATHS
IN LEVEL B
Command:
GETTING
STRONGER

1 BREATH
IN LEVEL B

1 BREATH
IN LEVEL A

... begins

1—1½

Command:
CONTRACTION
STARTS NOW

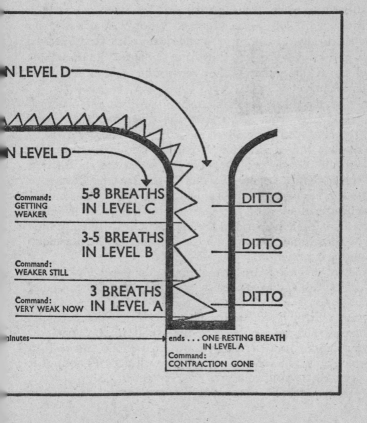

N LEVEL D

N LEVEL D

Command: GETTING WEAKER	5-8 BREATHS IN LEVEL C	DITTO
Command: WEAKER STILL	3-5 BREATHS IN LEVEL B	DITTO
Command: VERY WEAK NOW	3 BREATHS IN LEVEL A	DITTO

inutes

ends . . . ONE RESTING BREATH
IN LEVEL A
Command:
CONTRACTION GONE

As long as you breathe in each level carefully, maintaining a steady rhythm as indicated in Practical 2, you will do all of this without difficulty. In other words most trained women tend to provide too much rather than too little oxygen in their efforts to do the right thing. (See warning notes at the end of this chapter.)

Labour Diagram (3) will take you almost to the end of the first stage of labour. We shall learn how to handle the remainder in later lessons.

How to practise: You should use a helper for all labour-rehearsals. During rehearsal we try to create a situation which is as close to labour as possible by substituting appropriate arm and leg muscles for the uterus, and by using words as a substitute signal for the sensations which will be your signal or yardstick in labour of what is happening.

You should lie down in our basic position (see Practical 1) and have your helper use the diagrams. These have instructions on them which indicate to the helper when to say that the contraction is getting stronger or weaker. Naturally the helper also tells you when the contraction begins or ends. Labour Diagram (3) has a second alternative pattern because many women have noticed that this is what their uterus does and therefore this is necessary to maintain control. Your helper uses the instructions, to silently time you breathing and to indicate the changes in the mock uterine contraction.

The diagrams are based upon the average kind of contraction and have been worked out after observation of hundreds of women in labour. So they form a sort of basic 'recipe" which you use for rehearsals—but which you must adapt to fit your particular labour-situation. Don't try to fit your labour into the diagram but change the "recipe" (to which you will have then become well accustomed) as is necessary for your comfort.

While breathing according to the verbal signals you

should also check that only those muscles which you are using as substitute uterine contractions are contracted. Correct any inadvertent contraction of other muscles immediately. This is exactly what you must do during labour too—respond to uterine signals, breathe accordingly and check neuro-muscular disassociation.

Practise each Labour-Diagram once daily with your helper. Do Diagram (3) twice ... the alternative pattern needs practice too in case you need it in labour.

You can now discontinue the Disassociation Drill and its variations from Lesson 3.

Warning Notes:

(1) If you begin to find that you sometimes feel the need to take a big gulp of air while doing conscious controlled breathing this means you are contracting your chest muscles. Don't take in a gulp of air but blow out gently instead. You will feel yourself going loose inside your bra—a sure sign that the chest is completely relaxed.

(2) If you feel dizzy after controlled breathing you are overbreathing. This means too fast and too deeply. So make all your breathing somewhat more gentle and slow it down too.

(3) If you are trembling, the opposite is the case. Make your breathing somewhat more pronounced and the trembling will cease.

(4) If you have ever had convulsions—don't use *Level A* breathing during labour rehearsals or during labour itself but always start with *Level B*.

(5) In *Level B* and *Level C* make sure that the out-breath is more emphasised than the in-breath so that the chest is relaxed after each breath.

(6) Length of contractions given on Labour-diagrams is *approximate;* this means it's only a very rough guess, because *each* uterus during *each* labour develops a unique pattern for itself. Practise the basic breathing pattern on each diagram and don't try to fit it into the given length of contraction.

(7) During labour adapt these basic breathing patterns for each type of contraction to the special needs of your uterine function. If you have practised conscientiously this will come much more easily than you think.

(8) The intervals between contractions are *not* a good yardstick for measuring the progress of labour. Measure by the length and strength of contractions. This is much more accurate.

AND WHAT TO DO IN THE FIRST STAGE
OF LABOUR

IT is all very well to know how to work with the uterus, once it goes into action during labour. But you must also know how to work with doctor and midwife! You must also be very certain about "when" to go into hospital or call the midwife, and what to watch out for. So we will take a journey through the first stage of labour and put in the landmarks to simplify what you should know.

The pre-labour phase of thinning of the cervix is usually characterised by the weak, short contractions of labour diagram (1). These come at varying intervals; some women have contractions with varying pauses of 20 minutes, five minutes, ten minutes and so on, others have them regularly every ten minutes and yet others have regular contractions every three minutes right from the word "go". These intervals have no importance. It is the length of each contraction and its strength which in combination form an invaluable guide to your own assessment of progress.

During the last few weeks of your pregnancy you will have in any case noticed contractions of the uterus. At first it is not easy to distinguish them from the baby's movements, but after a while it becomes easier. These pregnancy contractions are a means of testing the ability of the uterus to carry out its job; they are also a useful opportunity to practise your breathing with the "real thing". You will soon find that even these gentle hardenings of uterine muscle are affected by your breathing and your control. The earliest contractions of the thinning of the cervix are very similar to these "testing" contractions. But they are also accompanied by certain physical and emotional "landmarks" which will help you to distinguish them.

The first landmark is the sensation of weak short

contractions. These contractions can be handled in Level (A) and are never longer than 45 seconds each. You may have a little note from your hospital or doctor or midwife which says "Come in to hospital, or call me when your pains (they mean contractions) come regularly every ten minutes". Ignore this! It's nonsense. The intervals between contractions are meaningless, as a way of diagnosing what is happening. Life would be a lot easier if they were. But there are some people who have thinning of the cervix contractions throughout, at three minute intervals but all about thirty seconds long. So these poor devils should obviously have been in hospital three weeks ago! The only way you have of diagnosing from your point of view (in other words without an internal examination) what's happening and how far you've got is by length and strength—the two factors combined. The important thing is whether the uterus is working, not the resting periods in between.

So during the thinning you have these weak short contractions. Frequently, particularly if they start at night and you are asleep, they are coupled with bursts of energy and excitement. This is one of the most noticeable emotional landmarks: and the urge to tell somebody!

Now, what do you do? You can't resist the urge for any length of time, worth mentioning. If this stage does start at night (it needn't, but it is quite common) this is what to do: Get out of bed and make two cups of tea, coffee, ovaltine or soup. This uses up some of the energy. And a hot drink is pleasant for you quite apart from comforting your husband for being woken up in the middle of the night for no good reason! Then sit and drink whatever you have made. If you now get a contraction you may realise that what wakened you was not in fact a contraction but simply a sudden wide-awake feeling. The contraction may be no more than you have felt in the past six weeks as part of your testing contractions, and you wouldn't feel very excited about that. But from now onwards while you are awake and even if you are still drinking your tea or whatever, put you cup down if you get a contraction and see that the body is completely decontracted while you are sitting there on the chair or the edge of the bed. Use just enough muscle power to keep your body upright and breathe in Level A. Do begin to handle the contractions *now*, while you are awake. Do *not* wait. Do *not* ignore the mild contractions and wait until they are painful. Because if you do this they *will* become very painful, and we won't want that.

But if when you have had your drink, the contractions are still just weak odd ones, don't spend the rest of the night leaping about like a mountain goat. Don't call the hospital. Don't call the doctor. Get back to bed. If you don't, you will eventually suffer great discomfort. It is vital during the thinning of the cervix that you spend as much time as possible asleep. I mean the normal period of sleep—and 2 o'clock in the morning *is* the normal period of sleep.

You may find that the excitement makes it very difficult to go to sleep at first but if you read for half an hour you will find that gradually if you make an effort to do the original decontraction drill just as a means of getting to sleep, you will sleep. Obviously you will sleep through the contractions instead of waiting to handle them. But while you *are* conscious and awake you handle each one.

For the remainder of the thinning if it continues during the day, you simply carry on as normal. You get up, you get washed and you get dressed. You do your housework. You don't have your husband sitting there with a stop-watch in his hand, waiting for each contraction. But every time you get a contraction, stop whatever you are doing. Lean against the nearest wall, mantelpiece, chair, kitchen table, sink, whatever it is, and breathe through your contractions. If by the afternoon it is still the same, go and lie down. Have a couple of hours rest in the afternoon and if you can go to sleep, all the better. If it is still the same by evening, go to bed early. Have supper, a hot bath and go straight to bed. If you can get two or three hours of sleep in before midnight, and you do go into labour later on, you will be that much better off. Because you will have already stocked up as it were, on rest. It is the worst thing you can do to go into labour proper—the dilatation phase—with the body tired and exhausted. This leads to an inefficient labour. So get as much sleep as you possibly can but otherwise carry on with your normal routine.

Gradually the following things will happen. Number one: the contractions will become stronger. And you will recognise this because you will find that breathing in Level A is not comfortable any more, and at first you might feel a bit puzzled But on the next one, start in Level A and as soon as you feel the greater strength you will hitch it up a notch into Level B. And if you need, go up to Level C. When you have done this for a few contractions you will realise that they are also longer, creeping up from 45 seconds to about 55 seconds. During the thinning, you had the odd ones of 10 seconds, 15 seconds, 30 seconds, 45 seconds, 25 seconds, they vary like this. But gradually as they get stronger, they creep towards a more or less regular length of 55 seconds to a minute. And for comfort you have to breathe during each one through Levels A, B, C, B, A and a resting breath. This will inevitably happen, sooner or later.

In addition two other things may happen. They may not happen at all or until much later, but if they happen now you must know, or you may worry. The first thing is something we call "a show". During pregnancy the cervix is plugged by nature with mucus to seal the uterus against infection. This plug comes partly away as a slight blood-stained mucus discharge. It must be slightly blood-stained to qualify as a show. You won't feel this but obviously you will see it. It is only a little. Whenever this happens all you do is write down on a piece of paper (which you should keep near the telephone where you will need such information)

"Show" occurred at . . . and the time.

Next the bag of water, or bag of membranes as it is called, may spring a leak. You will know this has happened if you suddenly find that you feel wet—it feels like suddenly losing control of your bladder! But it is only about a little thimbleful of liquid. Just put a sanitary towel in your panties in case you get some more. Don't put a sanitary belt on: this is much too restrictive.

And on the piece of paper write: "Membranes leaking at . . ."

If the leak repeats several times during the next few contractions, or if suddenly, in the middle of nothing in particular, the sanitary towel becomes very wet indeed, then the bag of membranes has burst. (This is quite different, the difference between two cupfuls of liquid and a thimbleful.) In any case now—and only now—is the time to *immediately* notify the hospital, or the midwife, if you're having the confinement at home. This is what you tell them: "The bag of membranes has burst now. I have been having contractions of . . . (whatever strength they were) for the last (however long it is)." If it is a definite leak or burst they will want to keep an eye on you, and in hospital if that is where you are going. They want to be sure that you're not wandering in the streets.

Now, none of this may happen until you are in hospital. In this case when your contractions have been this new medium-strong kind for about a half to three quarters of an hour, in other words when they have changed from Labour Diagram (1) to Labour Diagram (2) contractions and continued for half to three quarters of an hour, you do the following things: First, you can now be pretty sure that labour is established. Labour proper as opposed to the thinning of the cervix. So you have a bath. As hot as is comfortable for you, but not boiling! A deep bath—that means as deep as your bathtub and your tummy together will allow.

This bath is not for cleansing purposes. This is a bath to help increase the circulation of blood to your tummy and so make the transition from weak to medium-strong contractions easier to cope with. It is a very nice feeling lying in a bath and handling a contraction. By the way, you should *not* be alone in the house and the bathroom door should *not* be locked during this bath. A woman in labour must always be accessible at all times. Even when you go to the lavatory the door should be closed, of course, but not locked. So assistance can get to you should you need it.

While you are in the bath, someone should be cooking you a meal. Even if it is two o'clock in the morning. What you have will depend entirely on what you fancy. Your body will tell you whether it can cope with an egg, toast and marmalade or merely an apple. All we are trying to do, is, to stock up body reserves as they are needed. Otherwise you will go into labour, the available sugar in your blood will exhaust itself and you will get very tired—needlessly. In fact you will be starving hungry. But you won't feel hungry, simply weak. So this meal is therapeutic. And if your husband is going to hospital with you, for heaven's sake make sure that he eats too, because there won't be any restaurants. Many hospitals are in places where there aren't even any fish-and-chip shops.

If, when you are bathing or having your meal, you get a contraction, stop whatever else you are doing. Even if you are putting a forkful of food in your mouth, put it down. Lean on the table, handle your contraction, breathe and then pick up the fork again. If you are still having Labour Diagram (2) contractions or have slipped into Labour Diagram (3) by the time you have finished eating, now is the time to notify the powers that be: the local midwife if it is a home confinement, the hospital if you are going there.

By the way, if you are phoning the hospital, don't tell your obstetric story to the telephonist. Poor souls, they are very patient. But if you or your husband tell her all about your contractions, she will merely say, "Just a moment, I'll put you through to the labour ward". Then you'll have to start all over again. So do ask for the labour ward or maternity unit, whatever is the correct name in your hospital for this, and tell them. Tell them where you have got to: length of contractions, strength, if there has been "a show" or not, membranes intact or leaking. If the bag of membranes has just burst, tell them that first. Then it is time to call the ambulance if that is how you are going, or get out the car if you are being taken that way. Ask them to put you feet-first into the ambulance, by the way. It is much more comfortable to travel facing the engine than with your back to it.

When you get to hospital, or when the midwife comes, the procedure is pretty well the same. They will take your temperature and your blood pressure, they will feel your tummy—you know, exactly what they did the last, and goodness-knows how many times, you went to the clinic. They will then shave your pubic hair; this makes you feel a little bare and naked, but it is for hygienic reasons. You will be given an enema; this is a soapy infusion of warm water in to the lower bowel, so that it is emptied and there will be no resistance from a full bowel against the opening cervix. In Lesson 7 I will tell you how to handle an enema without all the discomfort that is normally experienced. You can have an enema so uncomfortably you feel you can't bear it—and you can have an enema during which you could be reading a book. This depends on you, not on the person administering it. Some hospitals don't use enemas now but use suppositories. These are simply things which look like little rockets which are pushed into the back passage. About twenty minutes later you have a normal bowel action. Then there may or may not be an internal examination. It doesn't matter whether you have one or not. By the way, if while you are being examined you ask "How far have I got?", most nurses these days will tell you. But some *still* draw themselves up to their full height and say "You wouldn't understand anyway, so what is the point of my telling you?" Well, this is very irritating. But it is not important, because what *you* do, doesn't depend on the examination but on what you experience. So what you do depends on what you feel, not on the fingers of the nurse or midwife. All the same, it is interesting to know and to satisfy your own clinical curiosity!

After this you will be left "to get on with it". This is the phrase always used. And the way you "get on with it" is as follows:

Now that you are in established labour, you must remain awake and alert between contractions. You can't be half asleep and suddenly come to, in the middle of a contraction, expecting to be in control of it. How you stay alert depends on many things—your preference among others. You may like to read, but if you like being read to, this is where husbands are invaluable. If it is daytime you can listen to the wireless, hospitals have wirelesses too. Some women are perfectly happy to sit there in bed handling their contractions and reading a book between times, with their husbands sitting there quietly reading too. I have seen this frequently. There are women who prefer to be alone. Either is fine. What is important is that you must be awake and alert. You *must not* try to sleep, once you are in established labour.

Handling contractions during this period is almost like a holy ritual. You handle each contraction with as much single-minded concentration and care as you can; in the correct manner, with the correct disassociation, with the correct breathing. Never, never, *never* answer questions during a contraction. If someone comes rushing in and says: "How are your pains, Mother?" when you are in the middle of Level D breathing you just ignore it. When the contraction has gone, then you can say, "I'm so sorry but I was having a contraction".

People will also come along from time to time to listen to your baby's heart—with a little silver stethoscope which you know well from your clinic visits. This is quite normal. You concentrate on handling your contractions, and maintaining alertness. (You keep yourself stimulated, in other words.)

Between contractions drink plain cold water whenever you feel dry. I'm going to give you a tip here. Buy yourself a little sponge. At Boots, on the counter where they sell real, not imitation, sponges. You'll find little bits of sponge which are sold for cosmetic purposes. You know, to put tinted foundations on with. It must be *real* sponge because this is tasteless. Ask for a saucer of water to keep near you. Soak the sponge in this so that it is wet, not dripping, but wet. After a contraction, take the sponge and pass it across the lower part of your face and mouth. You will find your tongue licking it and sucking it. This provides refreshment and emotional comfort. It is the equivalent of a dummy to a baby. And you may sit there thinking to yourself "How dreadful!" But labour is a very basic function. And basic physical needs make an alarming reappearance. "Good heavens" you may think, wanting to lick and suck things. Me, a grown-up. Just wait and see! One more thing. Your bowels will have been artificially emptied, so as not to leave a barrier there. But what about the bladder? Normally we empty it when we receive signals from it indicating that it's full. You know, one can always tell when one wants to "go and spend a penny". You *should* know by now—you've done nothing else for the past nine months! But in labour you very often don't feel the sensation which normally indicates a full bladder because of pressure from the baby's head. You don't feel anything even though the bladder is filling up. So it gets to a certain point of fullness, and suddenly you feel pain with every contraction. This is because the full bladder is in fact counteracting the opening of the cervix. To prevent this, you go and spend your penny

8

every hour. In labour you do it by time signals rather than by sensation signals as normally. No one is going to stop you—not in any hospital. They are perfectly aware that the bladder ought to be kept empty.

Occasionally there are reasons why women should stay in bed during labour. If this is so, you will be told; in this case you are quite entitled to ask for a bed-pan every hour. But you must keep your eye on the clock. If you find a little difficulty spending a penny, as you might well with all the pressure of the baby's head, if you are sitting there anxiously trying to do your best and nothing happens, don't panic. Just sit and wait. Have your feet firmly planted on the floor. Don't sit on the lavatory like most people do, leaning against the pipe or cistern behind you with your feet dangling in the air. Sit firmly planted. And handle your next contraction as you sit there. When the contraction has gone, contract and decontract your pelvic floor half a dozen times, and you will find to your amazement that this relieves the condition and your efforts will be crowned with success. Then you can smugly return back to bed.

All this is how "you get on with it"—until the nature of the contractions changes. And you will know it is changing because you can no longer handle the contractions comfortably with Labour Diagram 3. Then a completely different function will be taking place, the function which we call transition stage. Now you must do something quite different: in the next lesson you will learn what this different thing is; you experience the change in terms of sensation. But until then you just carry on.

Of course I have not dealt with all sorts of things that come in later—like the use of drugs, for instance. First we should get the physiological pattern of normal labour under our belts, so to speak. It is very important that you remember not to fix your mind on this pattern of labour too precisely. You should use what you know about labour, and adapt your knowledge to the special version of labour which *your* uterus will produce. Any preconceived ideas like: "It must be . . . because that is like the diagram" can threaten your control. Some labours have almost no relationship to the diagrams. For instance I remember one mother who sent us a labour report which said "Dear Mrs. Wright, my son was born yesterday. I'm sorry I can't tell you how long my labour was because I don't know. I was in the kitchen baking bread and suddenly I had a very strong urge to push. Five minutes later my baby was born". But such cases are rare!

B-DAY CONTINUES

THE stage of labour for which you will learn to breathe in this lesson is acknowledged by everyone concerned as by far the most tricky to handle. This is the TRANSITION STAGE. It is tricky even if you are trained, although even more difficult if you are untrained. Not, curiously enough, because the contractions are stronger or longer than before. On the contrary, transition stage contractions are usually shorter; they very rarely last longer than a minute and are frequently weaker.

But this isn't the problem, it's the fact that you frequently suffer—a word I can safely use here—an emotional change, and this is quite difficult to cope with. However, the more you know in advance, the less you will suffer from it because you will recognise it for what it is. It will be almost as if you are suffering it on the side of your face, while on the other side you will be grinning wryly and saying to yourself: "Oh, yes, *this* is what she was talking about!"

You will notice that the excitement you originally felt at the beginning of the thinning of the cervix begins to change when you are first handling contractions by going up into Level C breathing Labour Diagram (2) contractions. You begin to feel that you are terribly clever. Every trained woman does this. Although you don't actually say to people "Look how clever I am!" when you have first successfully handled a contraction and need to go into Level C, you will be thinking all the same, "Isn't it marvellous what I do." And who can blame you if you look rather smug? Then, when you get to Diagram 3, the-life-is-one-long-contraction bit, you are so busy that all your concentration is needed for what you are doing. It has been said that then women look as though they were taking part in a religious rite. It is just because you are concentrating completely. You will probably be quite oblivious when people come into the room and go out again. Even if the nurse suddenly grew two heads you would hardly notice. This is how it should be.

But in the transition stage your mood changes again. And it changes to what can only be described as irritability. The nervous system is handling two things at the same time and so it becomes extra irritable. It shows this in one of two ways. Regardless of how long you have been in labour you may suddenly feel desperately fatigued. You may have been in labour less than a couple of hours, but you will still feel "Oh I *wish* I could shut my eyes and just sleep through a contraction!" But, of course, it is fatal to do this. If you do, you don't remain alert, you don't calculate your breathing and the rot sets in. But the urge to do so becomes very strong. So it is mainly during the transition stage that you feel the need of someone else's support. Well-trained women just sail through the first stages of labour but even they find support desirable in the transition stage.

The other kind of queer emotional reaction will be the conviction that everything anyone does for you is wrong. Until then you will have accepted the ministrations of your private slave with undying gratitude saying "Thank you, darling! That was lovely": every twenty minutes. And all of a sudden whatever he does is wrong. He cradles your uterus for you, that's wrong. He lets *you* cradle it, that's wrong. If whatever he's doing, one way is wrong, even if he does it the other way it will still be wrong. Untrained women immediately begin to swear at their husbands when they get to this stage. Trained women have been known to swear, but at least not at their husbands. They just swear generally at the sad state of affairs.

You know, I have a private theory—and it is entirely mine, completely unsupported by the rest of the medical world—that the more control one uses normally (I mean if one is the sort of person who usually swallows and bottle's up one's feelings) the more violent by comparison is the outbreak in labour.

I will give you two examples which I rather like because they are classics in their way:

In one class we had a terribly nice girl, a sort of prototype "naice" English girl. She looked like an English rose, with a typical rose complexion and she behaved like one. Always terribly sweet, she just didn't get irritated, she didn't get upset, she was very philosophical, and if things didn't go in the way she wanted them, well . . . life wasn't going to come to an end. Ideal. I was with her during labour and in the transition stage. When she had finished a contraction she suddenly sat up in bed, looked me in the eye and said—she always spoke beautifully—"Oh, what a bloody bore!" She immediately apologised for what seemed terrible language to her—but I didn't think her words were all that strong really in the circumstances. Another nice example was a Japanese girl we had in class. She didn't speak any English. She just said "yes". And we discovered quite soon that she said "yes" to everything. She learned very well, all the same simply by mimicking. She, too, was terribly sweet and polite. If ever I showed her something and had to correct her I would say "No" and make her imitate me. When she caught on, she would always smile and bow, obviously saying, thank you. Well, during her labour she was doing beautifully; her husband was there too. She wanted him there naturally and so did we—he spoke English and we needed him as translator! During the first stage of labour when I wanted to tell her something I would ask her husband to translate. He would start the translation, then say "Ah, she understood that" and he didn't need to go on translating. So she must have picked up enough English to understand me during her nine weeks in class.

We got to transition stage, and the midwife went to fetch a trolley to take her into the delivery room next door. Her husband had gone out of the room for a minute, and I was left alone with her. When she had finished her next contraction, I explained to her that the baby would be born soon and that the midwife had gone to fetch the trolley. She quite obviously understood the sense of what I was talking about. But—she was in transition stage. And she looked at me all of a sudden and said: "I not hear Engliss now". After that, she would have nothing whatever to do with me. Every word I spoke had to be translated, for the first time during the whole of her labour. But when the baby was born not long afterwards she became terribly sweet and polite again.

This is what happens to emotions during the transition stage. I am not suggesting that you must control it; it is not under your control. On the contrary, I am simply telling you this is a part of this phase of labour. And at least it indicates progress. You don't feel it unless you are getting close to the second stage of labour. And the only way out of this is through it.

I always tell husbands not to argue with a woman in transition stage. It's useless. You might as well talk to a brick wall. You may even get to a point where on this emotional level you feel that the whole world is wrong, that everyone is treating you frightfully badly. If you do feel weepy, for heaven's sake have a little weep. Don't sit there swallowing it. If you do you will only feel more miserable than ever. I once said to a girl "Don't you remember? I told you about the transition stage?" "I know", she replied, "but I *still* feel miserable". On the other hand you may feel apprehensive—"Oh lord, I'm further on than I thought!"

Now transition stage sometimes only lasts for two contractions, in which case you won't get any of this. (You won't be very much in control of it either.) Two contractions worth of this peculiar stage you can cope with. But it *can* last an hour or an hour and a half. This is when your emotions play you up and this is when "through it" is the only way. I'm sorry labour is so awkward, but there it is . . .

One thing you must do. Once you are sure you are not dreaming, in other words that these sensations are not some figment of your imagination—notify the doctor or midwife. If yours is a home confinement, and the midwife has visited you earlier and gone away again, now is the time to get your husband to call her on the phone. Because the delivery is not far away and she needs to prepare her equipment. If you are in hospital, make quite certain that you ring the bell and tell whoever comes. But don't use the phrase: "I think I am in transition stage!" "I think I've started wanting to push" is the acceptable way of putting it. And you will see something interesting when you say this. The midwife or doctor will pull back your blankets and look at your pelvic floor with complete concentration as though you were going to produce rabbits out of a hat. It is strange to say the least of it. What on earth is there to be seen?

Well, this diagram shows what your pelvic floor looks like from outside -in other words when the blanket is pulled back. If your assessment of the situation is correct, and not just your imagination playing tricks, the baby's head will be back there somewhere in the birth canal or just settling into it. If this is so, the effect of the head at the top of the birth canal will be a slight movement of the vaginal walls at the height of a contraction when you are breathing in the One-two, One-two Blow! pattern. This movement is what the midwife is looking for.

Then, if you are *right* the midwife will get herself ready if you are at home and lay all her equipment out. In hospital you will usually be taken to the second-stage room or delivery room. Usually you are taken there either in a wheel-chair or on a trolley. I should remind you that you cannot sit up on a trolley. You'll fall off if you try. You will have to lie on your side when you are on the trolley in order to handle the transition stage contractions, otherwise you'll fall backwards. But in a wheel-chair you are in an ideal position because you are sitting up straight. And obviously you can handle your contractions as you go.

In most hospitals the second-stage room has just a bed in the middle. It is not like an ordinary bed in the sense that it is higher and the legs are taller, so that you are much higher up than you would be on an ordinary bed. This is so that doctors and midwives don't have permanent slipped discs

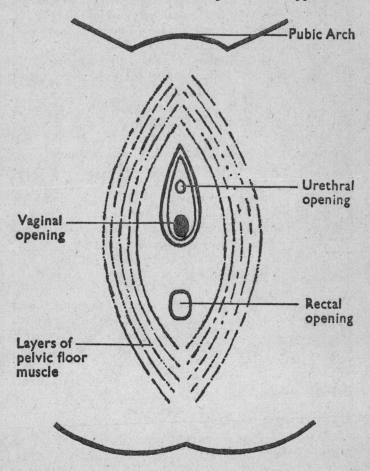

Pubic Arch

Urethral opening

Vaginal opening

Rectal opening

Layers of pelvic floor muscle

working down on the level of an ordinary bed. And instead of having springs underneath like an ordinary bed, it has a steel base. It looks more like a table made of steel, with a thick rubber mattress on top, which you will find very useful because it gives you good support when you get into the pushing or *expulsive* stage of labour. It is much more comfortable actually than an ordinary bed for this purpose.

Most hospitals have only one pillow on the delivery bed. You should ask beforehand to be allowed to take more pillows with you. Nobody should refuse you these days. You need support behind you in the expulsive stage of labour –for your own comfort.

When you get into the delivery room, please, please do not plead to be allowed to push. True enough, this urge becomes pretty strong. But do *not* ask: "Can I push?" You can never push too late. But you can with detriment, push too early. If any of the rim of cervix is left pressing on the baby's head, however thin it may be, this will be too soon to push. Then you are likely to be told "No" at first, which is rather disappointing. There are only two cast iron reasons for making your own pushing efforts along with the uterus. The first is when the pushing urge becomes really *completely* uncontrollable. It gets to a point where if Henry VIII were standing at the foot of your bed saying: "I will have you beheaded and put in the Tower if you push!" you would *still* push. It is quite irresistible. And that only occurs when the baby's head is sitting fair and square in the birth canal. This is fine. What usually happens is that a woman is handling her contractions, One, Two, One, Two and suddenly says "I'm sorry I just have to push!" Then they too will say, "Yes, that's alright!" The second alternative is this: The midwife, who has been watching your pelvic floor closely all the time says: "You can push with the next pain, I can see the baby's head!"

What is she talking about? What she means is this: at the height of the contraction she can see just a little of the baby's head through the opening of the vagina. This means the baby's head is sitting in the birth canal, so obviously what you have to do now is to go ahead and push. So when either of these two things happens you reorganise yourself at the next contraction for the pushing or expulsive state of labour.

In Practical 6 you will learn how to push. Now you may say of course, that millions of women manage to push their babies out without ever learning how. This is true. But there are efficient and inefficient ways of doing it. And we want to get maximum results from comparatively minimum effort.

I'm told by some mothers that I don't emphasise enough what hard work the expulsive stage of labour is. Oddly enough this isn't quite true. Hard work—yes. But not for you—for your uterus. The uterus does 80% of the work in pushing the baby out of your body. You do 20%. But *at the time* it feels as though you were doing 80% and the uterus only 20%.

If you want to have some rough idea of how much work will be done, look at the size of your sitting room. Imagine it has no carpet but just a wooden floor. Imagine you are a Victorian woman and with a bucket of lukewarm water, a bar of soap and a scrubbing brush, you are going to get this floor clean on your hands and knees. None of this TV commercial business with a modern mop and a detergent that whisks over the floor in 60 seconds flat. But real old-fashioned elbow grease. If you can imagine even faintly how much work this would take, then you have a rough idea how much work your body will undertake. Because as I said, 80% is done by the uterus. Even though it may not seem like it at the time, nevertheless it is true. So it *is* hard work. But it is satisfying work because you know you are getting places at last.

In a normal labour, when the baby's position is as it ought to be in the birth canal, if you push correctly the second stage of labour is painless. In a normal labour this is guaranteed. The first stage of labour we can't guarantee, but the second stage we can, as long as you do the right thing. If you don't, you can make it painful. And in fact the only wrong thing you *can* do is just that! I'll show you both ways. Then you can choose which you want.

The contractions in the second stage of labour are quite different from the others. You will feel two distinctly separate sensations. In each contraction, that is. By the way, just before I tell you what you feel, one word of comfort. If this is her first baby, every trained woman—I don't care if she is so well-trained that her training comes out of her ears—makes a mess of it for the first half-dozen contractions in the second stage of labour. Fortunately the uterus isn't very good at it either and it too makes a mess of it! So you don't achieve much between the two of you for the first half-dozen contractions. This is perfectly all right. Just don't get panicky. Women sometimes get terribly anxious: "After all that training I push when I shouldn't and don't push when I should!" Well, don't worry about it. Every woman does this. Half a dozen contractions-worth is wasted—except that it gives you time to settle yourself in.

The intervals between the contractions are also difficult. At the beginning of the second stage of labour you may well experience three, four, five, six, even seven minutes between contractions. Sometimes women get very worried about this. They think "Oh, my God—I'm going back to the beginning again!" But *you* won't do this I hope. You will use these intervals to rest.

Now the sensations are two distinct ones. The first one is a tightening around your tummy as the uterus gathers itself for its pushing effort. This is just a feeling that the whole thing is going tight, like putting on a very tight roll-on. And then the second sensation follows—it is not simultaneous. This is a very odd one, but very clear. You feel a bulge in your vagina. This of course is the baby's head. Now, I want you to imagine an object about the size of a Jaffa orange, in your vagina. Don't faint—just imagine it. Obviously this isn't something which happens every day, or even every week. Once a month might be a help because you could then get used to it. But you don't. You only feel this feeling when you've got the baby actually lying in the birth canal. And here the trouble begins—unless you know what you are doing. Instinctively you will try to tighten the pelvic floor against this bulge. You contract your feet and legs. This is bound to cause pain because the uterus is pushing one way while you are pulling the pelvic floor in the opposite direction. Inevitably this is going to hurt.

Now that you know how to make it painful, I'll show you how to make it painless. As soon as you feel the bulge, get clear in your mind the idea of pushing the bulge forward or out from your point of view. Because that is where it should be going! The easiest way to ensure that you do it is to remember to fix a visual target for yourself, somewhere in front of you. It could be the bed-rail, it could be Sister standing there, or her belt-buckle if you can see it. It could be a spot on the wall—it doesn't have to be anything interesting. Then decide to push the bulge towards it. Fortunately the human mind works in such a way that you can't think "Forward" and at the same time pull back. So if you think "Forward", you will work forward.

As soon as you encourage the bulge to move forward there is no pain. And it becomes a very satisfying activity because you *feel the bulge move*. You will push as hard as the uterus asks you to push. Now this is different for everybody; it is like asking how hard should you blow your nose? Well, nobody taught you how hard. You blow your nose as hard as your nose needs to be blown. In the same way, you push as hard as the uterus asks you to push.

You will hear all sorts of encouraging statements when you are doing this, from everybody. They'll say they can see the baby's head and tell you what colour the baby's hair is.

Don't fuss too much at this point about the colour of the baby's hair. They are looking into the comparative darkness of the birth canal, where the hair frequently looks dark when it isn't. But whether it's got dark hair or curly hair or no hair at all, at least it is very encouraging to know that you are pushing not just a sensation but a real something.

With each contraction, the bulging sensation becomes more. Finally, after about three-quarters of an hour, the crown of the baby's head emerges outside your body. The crown is the part of the head on which you would wear a diamond tiara or a bridesmaid's headdress if you were a bridesmaid.

Then we know that the next contraction after the crowning of the head will deliver the baby's head to below the chin. We know too that we want this to happen slowly. So this is one contraction when you will *not* push. But you do something else which allows the uterus to deliver the baby's head on its own without any effort from your tummy-muscles. This contraction takes about eight seconds.

When most people talk about "birth" it is these few seconds which are meant. They are not aware that everything which goes before, all this uterine activity, is all part of birth.

After this there is usually a pause of about a minute or so. Then you may or may not feel the next effort. If your baby has longish hair, you may feel it tickle as the baby turns inside the vagina. But you may not be aware of it. But if you do feel it don't shout at everyone "Stop tickling!" They are not there to tickle you, and their hands are usually occupied elsewhere. This is only the first of many situations where your child will be doing ticklish things to you. The baby may also cry; it is a very odd sensation, hearing your baby cry before you've even seen it, and you don't know whether it is a boy or a girl.

You may have to give a little help—a very gentle push

with the next contraction. This will deliver the shoulders, first the front shoulder and then the other one. Then the baby turns again. But you won't feel this because by now the birth canal is very stretched and there is no hair to tickle you. And the remainder of the baby's body just slides out virtually unaided by any deliberate effort. The uterus simply pushes it out.

Then you will see the baby lying there, still attached by the umbilical cord going in through the vagina and the uterus, to the placenta. And for the first time all your secret questions will be answered. And you know, you can't send it back now—either through the National Health Service or by a private doctor. In a couple of minutes you will see the cord being clipped about 2 inches away from the baby and again about the same distance away from you. Two metal clips are put on to act as tourniquets. Then the cord will be cut. When the cord has been cut, the baby is independent for the first time. (By the way there are no nerves at all in the cord so you don't feel anything.) The baby is usually wrapped in a warm towel or a sheet. And then it should be given to you, to hold.

I have no intention of telling you what you will feel when you first hold your own child in your arms. I can't tell you. Nobody can. There just are no words for this. But you don't need to be told because you will be fortunate enough to experience it. You will find all of a sudden that all the times you went through the lessons, all the weary months of practising and breathing and muscle-control and effleurage, will suddenly become in a way quite insignificant. Because all of a sudden you will have reaped the reward for all those months of patient work. You will hold this baby, towards whose birth you've done all that you could. This much you have; that whatever else may happen you have done the very best you could for your child And this right from the start is quite different for an untrained woman who sat hoping that someone else would do something. You haven't; you have prepared yourself. To the best of your ability, you have done the best that you could.

While you are sitting there reaping a just reward for all your efforts by simply looking at your child, the third stage of labour is happening, quite unknown to you. You don't feel anything; so sometimes it is easy to forget that the placenta is still in the uterus. Usually the placenta separates after the baby is born; the uterus and the placenta part company as it were. And one contraction delivers the placenta. In most hospitals you are simply asked to give a push They can see that the uterus has contracted, and is sitting on top of the placenta, by now in the vagina. From outside, this shows as a bulge in the abdomen. So they will say "Do you feel a pain?" meaning a contraction. And you will say "Er, well . . ." because it is so gentle by contrast with the strong ones which you felt before. In which case they will say "Alright come on then, give a push". Then you'll feel it sliding out.

In some cases the midwives and doctors like to push the placenta out themselves. Then you'll see the edge of a hand descend on top of your uterus. Now if you just lie there watching the hand on your uterus, you will feel the hand pressing in, then it will sort of spoon it out. This can be very uncomfortable because you will then contract your tummy muscles against it. So what you do instead is this:

If you feel the hand descend, go immediately into Level C breathing and push your pelvic floor slightly forwards. In other words you release it. Then you'll find that you feel hardly anything; in other words, you are almost unaware that something is happening. Certainly it is not painful. If you ask what they are doing, you will immediately contract your tummy muscles and pelvic floor and this *will* be painful. It takes about twenty seconds to push the placenta out whichever method is used: by hand or by your own pushing efforts.

The delivery of the placenta completes labour. You will

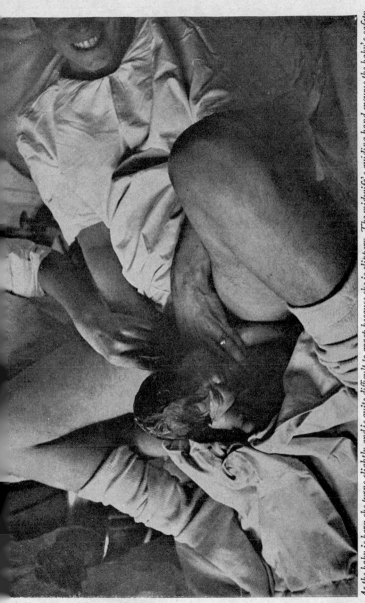

As the baby is born she turns slightly and is quite difficult to grasp because she is slippery. The midwife's guiding hand ensures the baby's safety

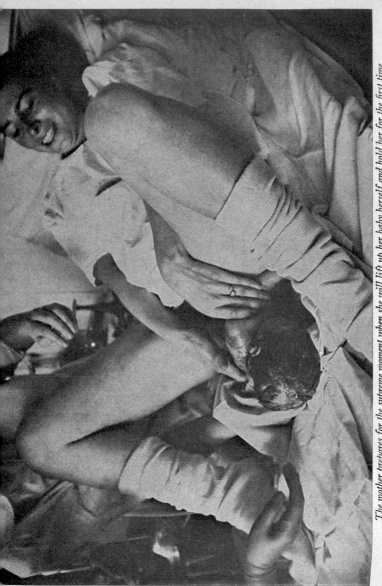

The mother prepares for the supreme moment when she will lift up her baby herself and hold her for the first time

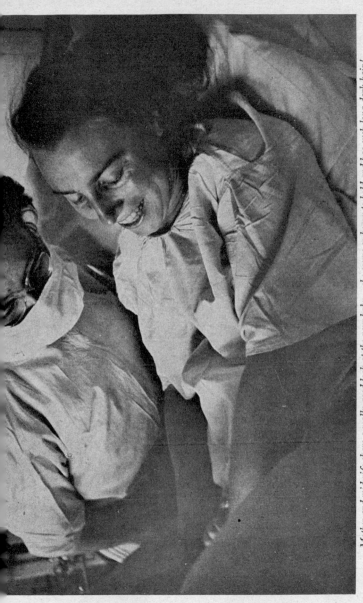

Mother and midwife share a really good look at the new baby – she seems so heavy to hold and has such long dark hair!

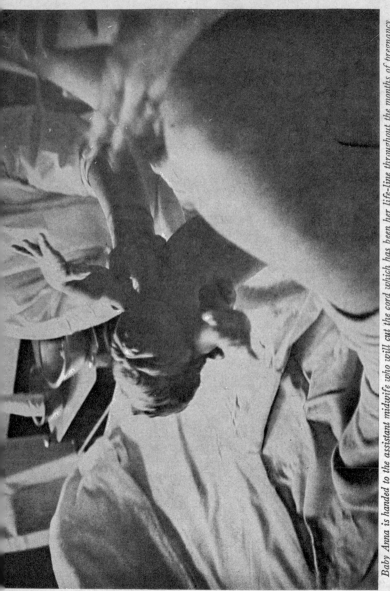

Baby Anna is handed to the assistant midwife who will cut the cord which has been her life-line throughout the months of pregnancy

find that you are bleeding, roughly as much as during a heavy period. So usually they give you, first of all, a perfunctory clean-up because your body is a bit messy, then they put two sanitary towels on. By the way, this will be the first time that you can use a sanitary belt. If earlier you were wearing sanitary towels because you were having a "show" you didn't wear a sanitary belt because it would squeeze the tummy and be uncomfortable. But now you don't have to keep the towel there by faith. So don't forget to pack a sanitary belt in your suitcase.

The next thing that happens to you is a cup of tea. If you hate tea, obviously you can have coffee; but whatever you have, it should be a hot drink with sugar, although not necessarily *in* it. If you hate sweet beverages, you should make up for the blood sugar which you have used during your efforts to produce your baby by taking either a couple of spoonfuls or a couple of dry cubes of sugar. Even better—because it is quicker—when you buy all the safety-pins and powder and things for the baby at the chemists before you come to hospital, remember to get one of those packets of flavoured glucose tablets for yourself. Give them to your husband to slip into his pocket. Don't spoil the flavour of your tea or coffee if you like it unsugared. But eat some glucose as soon as you can, to make up for that loss of sugar.

Now I have quite deliberately not told you anything about drugs. We discuss these in the next lesson. Nor have I told you about stitches, although you must have heard about them already. These are not strictly in the framework of a physiologically normal labour. This is a little bit extra and is not all that common. So this is something which we will learn in the next lesson too. After that, I discuss any variation from the normal because you must understand, just as midwives must understand, that every labour does not run like the one I have just described. And if it doesn't you must understand why not.

9

You can learn how you can best adapt yourself if it does deviate, by still doing the best you can under the changed circumstances. So first of all we get our normal "Textbook" labour clear. Then we add all the extra bits and variations.

DON'T PUSH YET!

YOU are no doubt becoming quite expert by now with your different levels of breathing, as well as in maintaining arm and leg muscles in contraction while at the same time keeping a weather eye open for any other muscles which might want to join in.

So now is the time to add another piece to the puzzle of how to handle "B-Day". First a little more about contractions. When I use the word "contraction" I mean just that. I am not pretending that it is really pain but we're not mentioning the nasty word! The uterus does contract; but muscles which are nearby, do tend to become involved with the tense activity of the uterus. This is what is painful.

It is rather like living in a house with a garden next door to another house with a garden. If your charming neighbours light a bonfire to burn their garden rubbish, you will get the smoke and soot particles over on your side, just as though you were having a bonfire of your own. So it is with the relationship between the uterus and the muscles of the pelvis.

The commonest "bonfire" effect happens in the tummy muscles. They often develop cramp-like sensations, at first only vaguely uncomfortable, but they can become acutely painful if nothing is done. Untrained mothers therefore often suffer quite needless pain which could be controlled if they knew how to help themselves.

Now what are we going to do about it? The pain is usually felt more or less along a horizontal line across the tummy, just where the pubic hairline begins. Just behind there, sits the cervix, and it is the sensation of the stretching of the cervix which reflects in the tummy muscles. For this you can do a strange kind of massage which has a French name—EFFLEURAGE. The equivalent term is BUTTER-FLY-STROKING. But I am not at all sure that Effleurage isn't simpler really. Anyway the name is not important. But doing this massage correctly is. It is vital that the massage is done with just enough pressure to avoid tickling, *but no more*. Any real pressure would irritate the uterus during labour and make the discomfort worse. Try stroking the back of one hand with the tips of the four fingers of the other hand. Stroke rhythmically, and don't tickle. It is a similar movement to stroking someone's temple when they have a headache. The effect of this stroking is to desensitise the skin somewhat; the underlying superficial muscles then relax and therefore greater comfort can be created. Effleurage can be done by you or a "slave" if you have one. If you look at the two diagrams, 19A and 19B (page 133), it will help you to practise it.

Practice is of course essential, because doing effleurage must become as automatic as breathing through the four levels. In fact from now onwards you should practise Labour Diagram 3 with effleurage. To do so will require you to use both legs as your "mock-uterus" in contraction, so that your hands are free to work. As you can see from the "effleurage" diagrams there are two kinds and you may use whichever you find easiest.

Effleurage Diagram 2 shows the second variation; this is also the one that should be used by the "slave".

4 Important Notes

(1) To be effective, effleurage must be done when the uncomfortable sensation *is* only uncomfortable—don't wait until it is really painful. It might be necessary to do it throughout the whole first stage of labour.

(2) It is important, too, to do effleurage only with the very tips of the fingers and to keep the rest of the hands away from contact with the skin-surface. Otherwise you will cause irritation, and not relief.

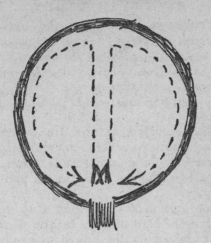

Diagram 19 Fig A

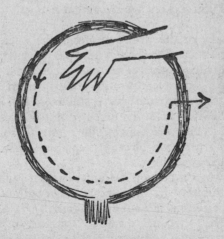

Diagram 19 Fig B

(3) You *must* do effleurage *throughout* the whole contraction with an even rhythm which remains constant, although your breathing-rhythm changes. When you need to breathe in Level D while doing effleurage, sing your tune in your head as before but do not, obviously, beat the rhythm with your fingers as well! Just maintain the rhythm of effleurage.

(4) If your husband is going to be with you during labour, have him practise effleurage during your rehearsal-session at the same time that you are maintaining the mock-contraction and the breathing according to the pattern on the Labour Diagram.

It is important to get accustomed to experiencing effleurage on your bare tummy. A little talcum powder should be sprinkled on the skin occasionally to avoid friction.

You will recall that you read in Lesson 4 how the contractions of the first stage of labour gradually change, and how you become aware of this change because the sensations you feel change also. What happens to cause this change?

The body of the uterus stretches the opening of the cervix until most of the baby's head has wriggled through it. But the opening is not yet quite large enough to release the baby's head completely—only three-quarters of it has slipped through with one quarter still to go. This is the phase of TRANSITION from the first stage into the second stage of labour. While still opening the cervix to complete the stretch, the uterus is already preparing for its expulsive efforts at the same time.

A few women do not feel any different sensations as a result of this change. In this case they continue to handle the contractions as in Labour Diagram (3). 70% of women do, however, become aware of pushing efforts made intermittently by the uterus at the height of the contractions during this stage. This intermittent pushing is at first very weak but gradually becomes stronger, until it seems to almost *demand* that one join in and make pushing-efforts with the tummy-muscles.

Until this time you will have worked throughout labour in relationship with your uterus, responding to its signals. So it would appear reasonable to also do this now and to make pushing-efforts when the uterus seems to demand them.

This Is Not So!

Now you will have entered the phase of labour, when you *must not* join with the uterus. Why? Because in doing so you may push the baby's head more firmly against the cervix; as well as causing you pain, this may possibly damage the delicate tissues of the cervix. Instead, you must now engage in an activity which will *detach* you from the activities of your uterus, so that you will neither accidentally interfere with its action, nor resist the signals from it. This activity is our *Transition Stage Drill*.

About 30% of women experience something else again. Instead of pushing urges, they find that the pattern of the contraction at its height becomes muddled. They feel themselves being pulled into this muddle and then they lose control. Should your Transition Stage pattern go like this, you too must engage in Transition Stage Drill to detach yourself from the muddle and remain firmly in control above it.

To summarise—whichever different pattern of signals occur in your labour, you deal with it with this special drill:

Transition Stage Drill

First change your position. Use whichever of two new ones illustrated in Diagram 20, Positions 1 and 2, you find most comfortable. In position 1 shown in Diagram 20 you

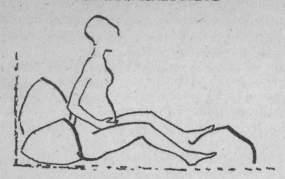

Diagram 20 Position 1

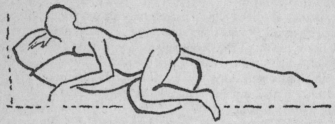

Diagram 20 Position 2

sit up straight, as if you were sitting on a rather wide seesaw, with your legs up on the plank in front of you. Push your buttocks well backwards, and use one or two pillows to support them. Leave the upper part of your back free. Bend your knees loosely and brace your feet lightly against a pillow in front of them. Practise what to do as in Labour Diagram (4) pages 138/9.

If you adopt Position 2 for Transition Stage Drill you have two pillows under your head and shoulders. Your underneath arm should be pulled forward to lie in front of your body so that the hand is on a level with your face. The upper arm lies loosely along the body. Put a third pillow next to your body and rest your "bulge" on it. The upper knee lies bent in front of the body on a fourth pillow with the underneath leg lying in an easy position behind.

To achieve the same pattern of activity as in Position 1 for transition stage, use your upper shoulder and arm like a rudder. Push it forwards—see Labour Diagram (4)—on the signal "Blow" and put it back into its usual position on the count of "one". Then repeat. This is also a useful alternative position for the first stage of labour.

Labour Diagram (4) indicates a repetition of the pattern 10 times. This is for practice only. During labour, you repeat the pattern as often as you need while the contraction is at its height, then you breathe in Level C as the contraction weakens again.

This may sound very difficult. But you should remember that we are deliberately *making* a difficult pattern, so that you must concentrate harder in order to detach yourself from the activities of the uterus. A firm upkeep of the rhythm of the pattern is essential if you want to stay in control of your responses. By the way, during labour you can change from one position to the other between contractions if you wish.

LABOUR DIAGRAM 4

TRANSITION STAGE—Cervix almost fully dilated-but don't push yet! Breathing includes 1-2-1-2-Blow pattern.

Note: On 'slump' purse lips to let air escape. On 'sit up' allow chest to take in air naturally, DO NOT take a deliberate breath. 1-2-1-2 is count, not a breathing rhythm. Count it in your head, as well as miming it with the lips, and tap the rhythm with your fingers on your leg.

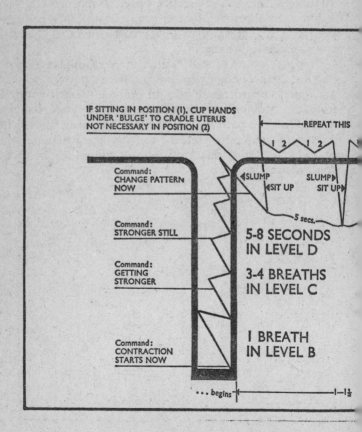

IF SITTING IN POSITION (I), CUP HANDS UNDER 'BULGE' TO CRADLE UTERUS NOT NECESSARY IN POSITION (2)

REPEAT THIS

1 2 1 2

Command: CHANGE PATTERN NOW

◄SLUMP   SLUMP►

◄SIT UP   SIT UP►

5 secs.

Command: STRONGER STILL

5-8 SECONDS IN LEVEL D

Command: GETTING STRONGER

3-4 BREATHS IN LEVEL C

I BREATH IN LEVEL B

Command: CONTRACTION STARTS NOW

••• begins

1—1½

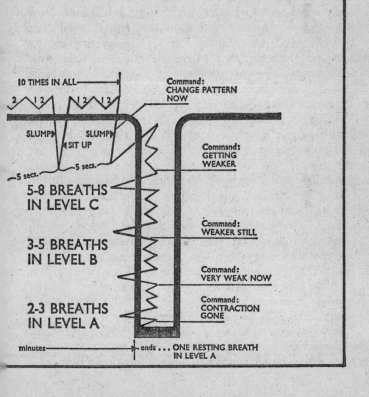

STILL B-DAY—WITH REINFORCEMENTS

FAR too many people spend far too much time during their pre-labour phase (long before they go to hospital, long before they even begin to think of the birth) without sleep.

This is not because they are in violent discomfort but because they are excited: having contractions is one way of passing the night. This is a very bad thing. They come to hospital already having lost a night's sleep; the body is already tired and so is that much more inefficient. Now obviously you can hardly call up the doctor in the middle of the night and say: "Look, I'm vaguely getting to the thinning of the cervix stage. Give me something to help me sleep." You will be very unpopular if you do. The best piece of advice I can give you is to get a prescription from your G.P. now. This will merely be a mild sedative, not a pain-killer, but literally just something to make you sleep.

Many people have something like this already because they don't sleep very well regardless of pregnancy. On the other hand if you have been sleeping like a woolly bear in hibernation until now, you may find suddenly that now you do need something. It is possible, with a little deliberate effort, to decontract all your muscles and so get yourself off to sleep. The contractions will not be strong enough themselves to keep you awake; but if you are already awake you will notice every one. This is quite unnecessary. And it is undesirable, because it makes the body inefficient. How can you function efficiently if you come to labour dog-tired? Far too many people still find themselves in labour thinking "If only I could sleep!"

Trained women don't usually need anything after that. But sometimes at about three to four fingers dilatation of the cervix, even in a normal labour, many women get a feeling not so much of pain, but that life really *is* getting a bit much! Not pain—that one can cope with. But now the contractions are coming so thick and fast there doesn't seem to be enough space between them to really collect one's energy again.

It's just like any real-life situation when you feel that life is too much for you: there is absolutely no reason at all for you to hang on grimly as though you were trying to prove something to yourself. Ask for an injection. You will only undermine your control of your own nervous system, if you lie there trying to perform unnecessary acts of heroism. The most useful injection is called *Pethidine.*

By the way, you should not go to hospital too early—and there is a very good reason why not. Some people still dash off to hospital at the first contraction; but they don't want you bouncing around in hospital any more than the midwife wants you bouncing around at home. Unfortunately though, hospitals can be somewhat overgenerous with sedatives and they might give you one with a longer lasting effect than is desirable. (Remember you will both want and need to be wide-awake later.) If you don't arrive at the hospital too early, this won't happen.

The effect of Pethidine if given at the right time—that is, when you are just beginning to feel that life is getting tough rather than when you are half-way up the wall—is that after about twenty minutes the whole pattern is tidied up and you begin to feel "I'm having a bit of a breather!" And this is just what you need: something to help you maintain your control rather than something to knock you out. Obviously you can't be in a drugged sleep and doing conscious controlled breathing at the same time! So you have something which will not send you unconscious but just help you to keep calm.

Pethidine will only make you sleepy if you are already exhausted when you take it. This is why it is so important to sleep during the thinning of the cervix; if you didn't do so at three to four fingers dilatation, you would be completely exhausted. It's up to you, really.

In the transition stage too, most trained women can manage without something extra. But not all. At this point one doesn't usually prescribe Pethidine because its effect wouldn't be felt until the second stage of labour and by then it would be too late. So what is usually offered is one of three different forms of inhalation gas. These are all capable of being taken by the mother herself; you will be shown how to use the mask. All three gases have the following effect: you will not be rendered unconscious but your sensory awareness will be cut down. So too will your control, if the gas is taken over any length of time.

For untrained women this effect is ideal because it is exactly what is needed. But for the best effect, the gas must be breathed in very deeply during the whole contraction, and this is what the nurses will also tell you when the time comes. But unless you have two sets of lungs, how can you simultaneously take deep breaths throughout the whole contraction and at the same time do your 1-2-1-2 Blow? Remind yourself of this if you are offered the mask as a matter of course. Nobody is saying "Take it—or else!"

But perhaps what will happen is the queer emotional state which I described in Lesson 5, and the associated muddled contraction pattern (see Lesson 5 page 116). In this case, it is not altogether undesirable to reduce awareness for a short time, to help one through a period of labour which can certainly be more uncomfortable sometimes than one wants to cope with. Twenty minutes of using the mask with deep breaths throughout each contraction may in such circumstances be of great help. Such a short period of inhaling the gas should not in any case undermine your subsequent control to any noticeable extent. But a longer period of inhalation might.

The effect of the gas is very similar to that of alcohol. Think of being in labour as very like driving a car in the rush hour; on one small whisky you could drive through the rush hour traffic without being greatly affected. But try drinking a whole bottle and see how well you could drive through the rush hour then! Well, up to twenty minutes or so of gas is your one small glass of whisky to help you face the rush hour. Any longer than that is like knocking back doubles. All you need to do is be sensible. Decide at the time if you want gas—and it can be a real extra help during a sticky patch—and then make proper use of it without feeling guilty.

You may again be offered the mask during the second stage of labour. This is because untrained women often resist when they feel the bulging sensation from the oncoming head and don't know how to push. But again, they won't insist that you have it. And all you need to do is say: "Look, can you leave it next to me on the bed and then I can use it if I need to?" This will keep everybody happy. You haven't refused their help, the container won't leak and you can't breath the gas by mistake without knowing about it.

This is fine. But the more wide awake you are in the second stage of labour and the more you are in visual communication with the midwife or the doctor who is delivering you, the more easily and effectively can you follow their instructions.

What else is likely to happen during labour to make "reinforcements" a good thing? Well, I'll now describe the five most common occurrences, and what is usually done about them.

(1) EPISIOTOMY. Have a look at the diagram on page 121. It shows what your pelvic floor would look like to the doctor or midwife during the second stage of labour, when the contraction is at its height. As you know, the pelvic floor is all muscle which gets thinner as the baby's head comes through the birth canal. This is just what we want,

this is the purpose for which we have been doing all these exercises. But one can never guarantee that the pelvic floor will thin sufficiently. And nobody is able to tell before the baby's head is born whether it is thinning or not. Even the person who is delivering your baby cannot tell until then. Or sometimes something else happens: the pelvic floor thins but overstretches—rather like old elastic. Naturally one wants to avoid both not stretching enough (which would mean that it might tear) and over-stretching (which would weaken it).

If either of these things occurs, an *episiotomy* is made. This is a small cut in the pelvic floor. In some cases, the doctor will give a small local injection into the pelvic floor, between the contractions. And then during the next contraction he makes this tiny cut. You will not feel the cut. But don't panic if you see a pair of scissors. What is being done is being done for the best—*your* best, because in the long run it prevents further weakening of the pelvic floor.

(2) ERGOMETRINE. When the baby's head is being born, you will usually be given an injection in your leg. This injection will be a drug called *ergometrine*. It will not put you to sleep. It has no effect on *you* at all. Its only effect is to make the uterus contract to prevent subsequent haemorrhage (prolonged heavy bleeding). And it is given as a precaution to almost everyone. All that happens is that a voice suddenly says "We're just giving you a little prick, dear!" Again, don't jump off the bed thinking "They've caught me at last! I'll be unconscious now for the next six hours". You will not be unconscious. It has no effect on your awareness at all. You may feel the contractions of the uterus and you may find, as some people do, that the contractions are a bit uncomfortable.

(3) STITCHES. If you have had an episiotomy, or if there has been a tear in your pelvic floor (you won't know about

this, by the way, if there is) then this obviously has to be repaired. This is done by *stitching*. If this happens this is how to behave:

You lie flat on your back with your feet supported in stirrups. (If you are having your baby at home you will be pulled down to the edge of the bed and your feet will be supported on two chair rungs.) This is to get your pelvic floor on a level with the person who is putting the stitches in. In other words, the doctor will sit on a stool facing you so that he can see to sew, just as you might in front of a sewing machine.

You will notice that first of all you get a series of small injections around the area to be repaired. Those will numb the area, although they will not take all the sensation out. You should breathe in Level A and decontract the pelvic floor. In fact the trick is to push the pelvic floor forward a little, so that there is no tendency to tighten the muscles. Push the pelvic floor away from you, continue to breathe in Level A—and you will hardly feel a thing. Go into Levels B and C if you still find you can feel too much. Keep the pelvic floor forward and *don't* contract your tummy muscles.

So your job, then, if someone is doing repairs to your pelvic floor, is to get up into your chest away from it—and let them get on with *their* job. Otherwise the more you try to "hang on" to your pelvic floor the more uncomfortable it becomes. And the more difficult it is, because of the muscle resistance, for the people to do their job at the other end.

These few stitches will take perhaps 10 to 15 minutes—no more. And there are pauses in between when nothing is happening; you can take a little rest and then the doctor will say "O.K.—now we're going to do another one", and away you go again. It may be uncomfortable. But it certainly need not be painful—if you don't contract your muscles. And you can see that your behaviour should be calm, co-operative and controlled—exactly as for the rest of your labour.

10

(4) AFTER-PAINS. After the baby and the placenta have been delivered, some women experience what are commonly called *after-pains*. This is the common name for the uterine-contractions which always follow labour, and during which the uterus is going back to its normal size. (You may hear the term *involution* used to describe this.)

For some women these contractions are painless, yet others find them quite sharp and unpleasant. Nurses often offer codeine tablets for relief but these aren't necessary. If you handle these after-contractions like a medium-strong labour-contraction they vanish after about half a minute.

After-pains commonly happen at the beginning of each feed at the breast for the first few days after the baby is born. Don't contract every muscle as soon as you feel the contraction, but continue to hold your baby gently and breathe as in Labour Diagram 2. Again, don't take codeine; it only becomes effective long after the contractions have passed. So it can't really help you.

Some untrained women spend the first two or three days after the birth of their babies in a permanent haze of drugs or discomfort. This is just not necessary.

(5) GLUCOSE. It is important to replace the large amounts of blood—sugar the body has used during its efforts to release your baby. Four ounces of glucose sweets, a packet of lemon flavoured glucose tablets or two tablespoons of honey eaten as soon as you get to your comfortable bed in the lying-in-ward will help to make you feel fit and if repeated daily for the first four days will help to cut down the emotional anti-climax feelings which many women otherwise experience.

(6) LOCHIA. After the birth of your baby, you will have a blood-loss rather like a heavy menstrual period. This will last for perhaps a fortnight. The official name for this is *lochia*. The sanitary towels you bring in to hospital should

therefore be maternity-towels rather than the ordinary soluble ones. (Ask your chemist for Size 3 maternity-towels.)

Although the bleeding will tail off after 10 to 14 days or even earlier, *you should not have intercourse during the six weeks following your baby's birth.* After six weeks you will have a post-natal examination from your doctor or hospital to make sure that everything has healed and the organs are back in place. After this you can safely resume sexual relations.

Practical 6

YOU'VE NEVER WORKED SO HARD IN YOUR LIFE!

IF you have worked through to this point as conscientiously as you should, your ideas about birth should by now be much more clear. And the picture of *your* role during your baby's birth should be forming.

No doubt the things you learnt during Practical 5 are still causing you some trouble. The Practical 5 work is the bit all the girls who come to our classes have difficulty with. Yet it *is* really simple.

All you must remember, is that your activity during the transition phase of labour is *not* related to that of the uterus. It is a separate activity designed to keep you occupied with a special movement and a special counting rhythm, while the uterus gets on with its own movement and rhythm. Your breathing throughout the special pattern is *natural* breathing, except for the "blow-collapse" bit each time.

The remainder of the pattern is a counting rhythm while breathing goes on. Don't forget to mime your counting with your lips all the time you are doing it; this habit will assist your control when the pattern comes into use during actual labour.

Now at last you can learn what to do when the midwife or doctor says the magic words "You can push now!" Remember the golden rule which says that you can never push too late but you can make labour very painful and do damage to the cervix by pushing too early. This is why you must be as patient as you can at this point during your labour. But when you are told that you can now push with safety—then you must know exactly *how* to use your pushing efforts to best advantage.

Practise in the following position: Lie flat with a soft

cushion under your sacrum, so that your body is quite horizontal below the waist. Above the waist have three to four pillows arranged in such a way that you are leaning against them as though you were in a deck-chair. Plant your feet flat on the floor with the legs as wide apart as possible. Check that you are not sitting on any part of your pelvis floor.

Next, try out the position for pushing. Tuck your hands behind your knees, and hold your elbows well out. Now *lift*

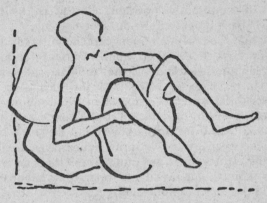

Diagram 21

your legs in that position, so that your feet dangle loosely off the floor. Put your chin on your chest and tip your shoulders forward off the pillows. Think of this as an attempt to touch your knees with your nose and this will help you to understand the position better. But don't make the mistake of trying to do the opposite and bring your knees up towards your nose instead—this tightens the pelvic floor and becomes very uncomfortable for your chest.

When you are experimenting with this position it may

strike you as very undignified and strange. If so, you might remember that it is derived from the natural squatting position for childbirth used by primitive women: they do this instinctively because it is the position in which the vagina expands most effectively. *But* primitive women also squat like this when they peel yams or grind corn. So it is an easy position for them, and one to which they are accustomed. Your body and mine are not used to squatting; we should certainly fall over after a few moments if we tried to sit in this position. And we should certainly not be able to make active pushing efforts! So we have a compromise version of the primitive position, allowing us to also have our lower back supported and our feet dangling.

Now that the position no longer seems quite so odd, let's find out how to use your tummy-muscles for pushing. During labour, the pushing efforts should be made when the uterus is pushing too. You will feel this as a strong urge—very similar to the feeling when you are about to have a bowel-movement. But it's not in the same place, because the vagina is in front of the bowel and there is a layer of muscle between the two. During rehearsal you will only make the efforts with your tummy-muscles as an exercise. The combined tummy-uterus operation happens only during the second stage of labour.

To make sure that you know exactly what you are doing with your tummy-muscles and so you don't do the wrong thing by mistake, do it deliberately now.

Then you will feel the difference between right and wrong efforts at once.

(1) WRONG EFFORT. Put your hands over your tummy just above your pubic arch. Now pull your tummy in as far as possible, as though you were trying to touch your backbone with it. Notice how the pelvic floor comes up and the whole area feels tighter than ever before. The openings in the pelvic floor feel smaller as well. Now let your tummy-muscles relax.

(2) RIGHT EFFORT. Put your hands over the same area and try to push them away with your tummy-muscles. At the same time push your pelvic floor forwards. If you can feel a sensation of "wanting to spend a penny" or just a loosening of the vaginal opening then you are making the effort correctly.

Experiment with this effort until you are aware of a definite sensation in the pelvic floor and not just in the tummy-muscles.

With the position for pushing and the pushing effort itself sorted out, now all we need is to add the breathing-drill. Do you remember Exercise 6 in Practical 2 for the breast-muscles and the special breathing exercise with it? (Check it on page 55). This breathing-exercise really belongs with the pushing-efforts for the second stage of labour.

You will find in labour that each contraction of the pushing-stage begins with a tightening of the tummy-muscles lasting about 8-10 seconds and followed by the pushing-feeling. You follow what the uterus does. In other words, you make pushing efforts when it makes them and not otherwise. So when you practise, this is what you do:

(1) Take your first two breaths in Level A while positioning yourself in the pushing-position.

(2) Take in the third breath and hold it.

(3) Put your chin on your chest, push your shoulders and ribs downwards and, still holding the air in your chest, push your tummy-muscles and your pelvic floor forwards as you just learnt to do.

(4) Hold this while "blocking" the air in your chest for about ten seconds.

(5) Raise your chin, gently release what air is still left in your chest, and hold the pushing-position while you do so.

(6) Now take a new breath in Level A, "block" it again and repeat the pushing effort.

After the second "block-and-push" cycle, release the air again, and lie back against your pillows as *delicately as you can.* If you feel breathless, breathe in Level C until you can breathe normally again. It is most important that you remember that there must be a marked contrast between the primitive thrust of your pushing-efforts and the slow grace of a Victorian lady with which you recline against your pillows. This slow, graceful movement is very necessary; the baby's head slides back a little after each contraction and when untrained women fling themselves back, panting wildly after their efforts, the head only goes back even further.

The second stage of labour has been compared by some people to a boxing-context, with the pushing-contractions as the rounds, and the rest as the periods between the bell when the boxer goes back to his corner. He does this to rest—and so do you, between each round of contractions. Like the boxer, you may use your sponge or take sips of water just as you need.

The average contraction during the second stage of labour lasts about 30-40 seconds giving you enough time for the drill described. But if you make too long pushing-efforts during your labour for each second-stage contraction, yet still feel some pushing-urge, just repeat the block-and-push pattern for a third time, going into the "Victorian lady" routine at the end of each contraction and taking resting breaths in Level C.

Labour Diagram (5) (pages 154, 155) repeats the practice-instructions; your daily practice should now include one run of this block-and-push drill. You can also do Exercise 6 from Lesson 2 without the breathing-drill, as you are now practising with your pushing rehearsals. Notice how the pattern of muscle-contraction and relaxation has changed. For Labour Diagram (5) your face, neck and shoulder muscles are contracted, as are arm, chest and tummy-muscles. Yet, *at the same time,* the muscles of your pelvic floor and legs are completely relaxed.

On the labour-bed you will position yourself exactly as

you are lying on the floor, but you won't need the little cushion under your sacrum. Ask the midwife to allow you to have several pillows behind your back as you are pushing. It makes the job so much easier—and you will be grateful for anything that does this. Remember that during this hour or hour-and-a-half, you will be working as hard as any trained athlete in a race—or as hard as the Victorian woman who had to scrub her floor *and* recline with ease!

LABOUR DIAGRAM 5

SECOND STAGE OF LABOUR: I—Uterus pushing baby along birth canal: Now breathing pattern to include:

Block-and-Push Technique

Take a breath in Level A and hold; put chin on chest; push shoulders and ribs downwards; push tummy muscles and pelvic floor forwards.

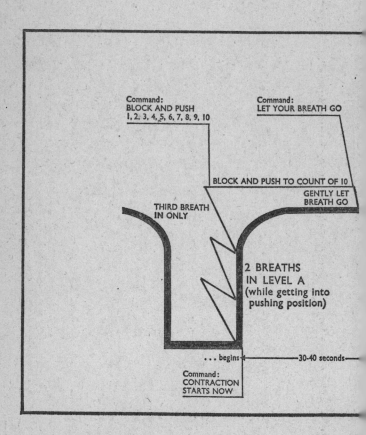

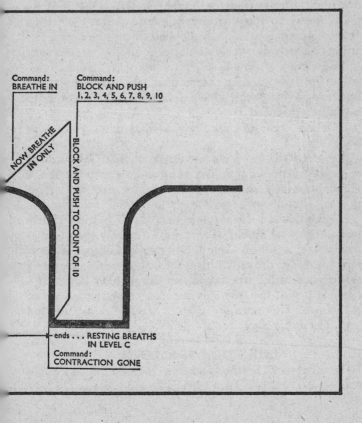

Command:
BREATHE IN

Command:
BLOCK AND PUSH
1, 2, 3, 4, 5, 6, 7, 8, 9, 10

NOW BREATHE
IN ONLY

BLOCK AND PUSH TO COUNT OF 10

ends ... RESTING BREATHS
IN LEVEL C
Command:
CONTRACTION GONE

WHAT IF IT ISN'T LIKE THE TEXT BOOK?

So far something we have never discussed is a situation that can happen to any pregnant woman: for reasons that neither she nor anyone else can control, the labour does not progress physiologically in the way that it should.

Now that is a fact that you should face. There *are* certain known variations from the normal pattern. One of these might happen to you—just as it might happen to me too if I become pregnant again. I don't want you to be needlessly anxious about this. It's much better to be fore-armed with the knowledge of how to adapt to any of these variations, just as you would adapt to normal labour. So there are certain procedures which have to be undertaken in order to normalise a situation like this.

What are these procedures and what must you know about them?

The first variation from the usual course of labour, and by far the most common, is that for some reason the uterus will not start its labour mechanism working, even though, as far as the doctor can judge, it ought to.

Judging this is not a matter of that "date" (which is fairly inaccurate anyway) but of examining the way the tummy-muscles are, and how large the uterus is. Factors like the apparent size of the baby's head and its position in the pelvis will also determine whether labour should have begun. If it does not begin, the uterus is encouraged artificially to go into labour. There are a number of ways of doing this and they all go under the heading

INDUCTION OF LABOUR.

The most usual methods used in Great Britain at present are:

(1) OBE as it is commonly called in midwives' jargon. Unfortunately this has nothing to do with going to Buckingham Palace in a new hat and being presented with a medal! These initials stand for Oil (Castor), Bath and Enema, which are given to the expectant mother in that order.

It will be obvious to you that this is an attempt to stimulate the uterus into action by actually stimulating the bowel which of course lies just behind it. The only thing about an OBE which is somewhat unpleasant is the Oil. Castor oil does not taste nice. However, the following recipe will make it somewhat less unpalatable:

If you go into hospital for an OBE, take with you a small quantity of Bicarbonate of Soda in a twist of paper and a bottle of concentrated fruit squash. Ask the nurse who brings you the glass of castor-oil for a large empty glass and pour about an inch of the undiluted squash into it. Pour the oil on top and follow this with another inch of squash. You will see that these two substances don't mix but that the oil sits between the two layers like the filling of a sandwich. Now add a teaspoon of Bicarbonate of Soda and stir. Drink the mixture while it is still fizzing. You will find that this way it is almost pleasant to take.

For the enema, refer back to the drill for repair of episiotomy in Lesson 6 (see page 145). You should keep your pelvic floor disassociated and breathe in Level C throughout the few minutes it takes to give it to you. You will have plenty of time to get to the toilet! People always panic and think that they cannot retain the liquid but actually you can easily do so if you keep calm.

An OBE may or may not get you into labour; but apart from a short period of discomfort while you are in the toilet, it will not alter the pattern of labour in any way. If this is not used, the next line of approach is usually:

(2) ARM. The initials stand for Artificial Rupture of Membranes. ARM is always done in hospitals and always by

a doctor. Again it is almost unnoticeable by you—if you follow exactly the episiotomy drill described in Lesson 6.

It takes just a few moments; then you wait for labour to begin. This may happen within 20 minutes or within a few hours or even not at all. However, the pattern of labour is usually unchanged except that the doctor may also stretch the cervix a little whilst he is rupturing the bag of membranes. In this case you can begin your labour with Diagram 2 contractions rather than with Diagram 1. Sometimes the doctor will merely loosen the membranes from the cervix and this will be enough to start labour.

Incidentally "dry" labour does not exist, except in old wives' tales. It cannot because the placenta replaces the fluid in the bag of membranes about every three hours and goes on doing so until the baby is born. In any case *all* the water in the bag does not drain away but only that which is able to leak past the baby's body. The rest usually follows the baby like a warm showerbath after its birth.

(3) ORAL "PITOCIN" INDUCTION. An alternative method which is coming into fashion now is to give the expectant mother small sweets which are dissolved in the mouth by holding them between the upper gum and the lip. These sweets contain tiny amounts of a hormone which stimulates uterine action. This is not unpleasant; but it does take a while to obtain the effect of stimulating the uterus.

(4) DRIP INDUCTION. Some doctors prefer to give this hormone by diluting it with a sterile salt-solution and passing it into the vein of the arm or hand over a period of several hours.

(5) FORCEPS DELIVERY. Sometimes it is necessary to assist the baby out of the birth canal. This can happen if the baby is simply taking too long to emerge, or if it is lying in the breech position and extra help is needed to get its head (which of course comes last) out of the birth canal. This is known as an *instrument delivery* or a *forceps delivery*.

Unfortunately these are nasty jargon words which, as you

know, can conjure up the most terrible and frightening ideas. But a forceps delivery is basically quite a simple thing. The obstetric forceps themselves look rather like the kind of tongs one uses for serving salad or for lifting clothes out of a washing machine. Obstetric forceps in fact do a similar job. Only they are made of metal, as wood or plastic could not be sterilised so efficiently.

Each blade of the forceps is about the length of a hand. So the two blades form two metal "hands" to hold your baby's head. Attached to the forceps are long, hinged handles and these remain outside your body. With these, the baby is pulled along the birth canal from below instead of being pushed from above. And that is all that happens.

The sort of situation in which you would have a forceps delivery might be something like this: you have been pushing for, say, an hour or so. But although you are pushing very well, there isn't much progress. This isn't because you aren't doing it well, but because the baby just persists in sitting there in the birth canal. Normally one doesn't leave the baby there for much longer than that. If its heartbeat shows, when it is examined, that the baby is getting tired, this is a sign that a forceps delivery is advisable.

Equally, if you yourself were terribly tired for one reason or another and you weren't pushing very effectively—not because you didn't know how but because you just couldn't—then obviously a forceps delivery would help both the baby *and* you.

From the baby's point of view, the only difference between normal labour and a forceps delivery is that he is being helped and every possible precaution is being taken to see that he doesn't damage his body during this difficult job—especially if the delivery is a somewhat rapid one, following as it often does on such a long period of sitting in the birth canal.

Some forceps deliveries are done under local anaesthetic, in other words the pelvic floor is numbed. In this case you would be as conscious as you are now and your behaviour should not differ from the usual pushing-drill and you would push with every contraction. You might perhaps have to be told when your contraction began; someone would keep their hand on your tummy and say "All right—push now!" Then you would breathe in and blow, breathe in and blow, breathe in and block-and-push, just as before.

The only difference would be that you would feel the bulge of the baby's head moving much more quickly along the birth canal. Obviously, for you would be doing only half the work. This is to be expected—and is perfectly all right.

But most forceps deliveries are done under a general anaesthetic. So for a period of about 20 minutes you would be fast asleep. But it *is* only a very light anaesthetic. And you know, if you were having a rough time during your labour, you might find it rather pleasant to be helped to sleep—and then wake up to find it was all over and you had a beautiful baby!

You may ask, "What can I do to prevent a forceps delivery?" The answer is, nothing. Sometimes it just happens that the uterus has got the cervix to full dilatation, the baby's head has slipped through into the birth canal, and you are told "You can push with the next pain". You push—and nothing happens.

I knew of a case like this. The mother arrived in hospital fully dilated. They took her into the labour ward straight away. "All right," they said, "After the next pain you can push!" What happened? Her contractions began to get weaker and she had no pushing urge worth mentioning.

Why the uterus behaves like this, heaven only knows! Sometimes it is too tired; but sometimes it can't be this. This woman's uterus had been in labour for only three hours, so it could hardly claim to be exhausted. Sometimes the baby's head cannot emerge from the bony pelvis because of the way it is positioned and you just can't push it out.

Note: cot nursing. Whatever the reasons for a forceps delivery may be, you will certainly appreciate that it indicates one thing; that the baby has been having a somewhat rough time—much rougher than normal. And so when a baby is delivered this way, every hospital follows the practice of *cot-nursing* the baby for 24 to 48 hours. You will not be allowed to hold the baby—nor will anyone else. It is not breast-fed during that time. It is both fed and changed in its cot. It is not bathed either, just washed right there in the cot.

Unfortunately one is very often not told why this happens. One is simply told "I'm sorry. You can't see your baby." But you *want* to see your baby. Everyone else's baby appears. Why not yours? But "You won't be able to see your baby" they tell you, "until the day after tomorrow!"

Well, mothers always assume the worst. But you know, there isn't any "worst". The only reason why the baby is in this cot is so that he won't be tossed around. It is to give the baby ample opportunity to have 24 to 48 hours of complete rest. This is why the baby must be alone.

So instead of getting all upset about it, recognise that it is done as a safety measure and not as a means of being cruel to mother or to baby. You can make up afterwards in terms of cuddling for what the baby is missing during these 24 to 48 hours. And if you get into a state bordering on hysteria, you won't be much use as a mother when you *can* hold the baby! You will also affect your milk supply. So don't do it.

One London teaching hospital, as well as allowing the mothers to get up the day after the baby is born, has castors on all its cots. In fact the cot stands right next to Mum's bed. So Mum can see her baby but she can't pick it up. If the baby needs feeding, it is given a very weak milk solution—in the cot by her. She can't cuddle it. But she can see it just as much as she wants. Nurse comes and takes the cot away to wash the baby, and then brings it back again.

But in some hospitals babies are kept permanently in a

nursery, and the mothers are not allowed out of bed for four days or more. Then you can't do this. This is a safety measure. But it is a very sad one.

(6) CAESAREAN OPERATION. One other thing which can happen to anyone and everyone is that even with all the best intentions in the world, the delivery of the baby is just not possible through the normal channels.

For instance, if you had been in labour for about two days and there had been little advance in the dilatation of the cervix, the baby would feel the strain, and undoubtedly so would you. Or sometimes the placenta slips its moorings and there is much more bleeding than usual. One doesn't wait and see in these circumstances. On does a *Caesarean operation*. This means that an opening is made into the uterus through the wall of the tummy. The uterus then delivers the baby into the doctor's hand instead of into the birth canal. Sometimes too, the mother's pelvic outlet may be too small to allow a baby of normal size to pass through. So this would also be a situation to make a Caesarean operation necessary.

If at any time during the first stage of labour the baby's condition indicates that it is not happy about what is happening (and a very careful watch is kept all the time) then this would be another situation when a Caesarean operation would be performed.

There is another situation too—and a very dangerous one.

You should let your doctor know *immediately* if this happens: if at any time between now and the time you either go into hospital or have the midwife come to your house, you notice that you are losing fresh blood. By "fresh" I mean a bright red loss and not the bloodstained discharge called a "show". It is always safer to notify him unnecessarily than it is to not do so.

Bleeding during pregnancy often is a sign that the placenta is becoming detached, and this, of course, must not happen until after the baby is born. If it *does* happen, this is an urgent situation. And it needs the specialised skill of your doctor and midwife; they have the experience to decide what is to be done.

The whole of Lesson 7 sounds as though no one ever had a baby born naturally as it should be, doesn't it? Of course you realise that this is not so. But having extra knowledge about things which could happen—even though they actually happen quite rarely—will help you to understand any situation which is not usual. It will help you, too, to recognise when intervention by doctor and midwife is necessary.

You should also be aware that you are not in any way able to prevent these variations from the normal pattern of labour. But everything you can do to help yourself stay calm and co-operative benefits both you and your baby in the end. Perhaps Lesson 7 is your most useful weapon in a way: use it to fight any horror-stories your friends might whisper to you. Knowledge of all the facts rather than misunderstanding of a few fragments is an excellent protection.

NOTE: If your labour does involve any of the above variations you should remember the Golden Rule which you already learnt in Lesson 6: whenever any doctor or midwife is working in the area of your pelvic floor, decontract your tummy muscles and pelvic floor muscles, get up into your chest and breathe in Level C. This obviously applies to all internal examinations, enemas and similar procedures.

SOME EXTRA WEAPONS
IN CASE OF NEED

YOU may remember that at the end of Lesson 6 I said we
would learn about the handling of labour if it did not follow
the usual pattern. The commonest variation is BACK-
ACHE-LABOUR.

This type of labour is so different from the usual pattern
that many women are not even aware that they are in
labour! They only feel an intense and very uncomfortable
backache. However, if it should happen in your case you
will find it easier to recognise if you realise that you can
apply Labour Diagrams (1), (2) and (3) to your back, as it
were, instead of to your tummy.

By now you will have experienced "testing-contractions"
in your tummy and you will therefore be familiar with the
wavelike pattern of sensation which is shown on the labour
diagram. Perhaps you have even begun to "see" the
sensations as a labour diagram picture. Well, just think of
this as being in your back rather than in your tummy—then
you are half-way to recognising backache labour.

The breathing and disassociation drill for handling the
contractions is exactly the same as for the more usual
discomfort in your tummy. But with backache you cannot
lie in the usual positions—it would be too uncomfortable.
And as backache-labour is usually caused by the way the
baby is lying in the uterus, we must try also to help it to turn
as well as deal with the pain which results from its unusual
position.

The rules for handling backache labour are very definite:
1. All pressure must be taken off the back
2. The uterus must be tipped forward during contractions
3. The uterus must be supported during contractions

4. Back massage or back-effleurage can be applied during contractions
5. Position should be changed about every half-hour to keep up the morale
6. Between contractions a cold compress over the sacrum is a wonderful boon.

NOTES:

(i) *Change of position*

A backache-labour tends to have a longer first stage than an ordinary one and the frequent continuing ache between contractions hardly helps one to keep cheerful during this time. A change of position is very useful because a change in this case is "as good as a rest". You will usually find that a change of position every 20 minutes or half-hour is just right.

You will find four different positions described in this chapter, which women with this type of labour have found especially beneficial, but essentially any position which is comfortable and allows you to breathe correctly, is satisfactory.

(ii) *Cold compress*

It has only very recently been found that a cold compress along the length of the sacrum and lower spine almost completely gets rid of the continuing ache if applied between contractions. Your own face-flannel, wrung out in cold water (ice is an added help) and folded into a small polythene-bag will do the job perfectly. (The polythene-bag prevents the sheet from becoming wet.) The compress should be taken off during contractions while back-massage or back-effleurage is applied.

(iii) *Back massage*

This *can* be done by you if you are alone during labour. But it is a real help to have your husband use it instead, because this allows you more rest. But it has to be practised, by him as well as by you. When practising it, use a practice contraction from Labour Diagram (3). While you are breathing correctly, according to the helper's instructions, he fixes his thumb on top of your hip-bone, as far back as he can. If you lean towards the side on which he is about to massage he will find the right spot more easily. With the thumb fixed, his hand should move in a fan-like motion from your spine towards the edge of the hipbone, kneading the muscle firmly and rhythmically. (Think of preparing dough for breadmaking and you will get the right kind of movement.)

The massage must continue throughout the whole contraction in order to be effective. It can be done on either side because there seems to be a reflected relief on the opposite side as well. So one-sided massage is enough—and it conserves your helper's energy too! Some women seem to find that *effleurage* done along the sacrum and lower spine is more effective than back-massage. Others find alternate massage and effleurage best. As long as you and your husband become skilled at doing either form of massage, you will find the best combination for your particular labour fairly easily.

(iv) Position for backache labour

The diagrams following this paragraph illustrate clearly the four positions. Practise with the Labour Diagram handling contractions in each of the four positions.

Position 1. This is particularly useful in early labour. (First stage or even during the pre-labour phase if backache occurs.) Sit on an ordinary wooden chair. Don't lean against the back of the chair, but sit halfway along. Put your feet firmly on the floor in front of the chair. During contractions lean forward, resting your forearms on your thighs. Notice that this takes pressure off your back and also tips your body—and therefore your uterus—forward. The thighs act as supports to the uterus rather like book-ends.

Position 2. Put a cushion on the floor in front of a chair and a second cushion on the chair seat. Kneel on the cushion on the floor facing the chair and keeping your knees slightly apart. Lean forward and rest your forearms flat on the cushion on the chair. During contractions, lay down your

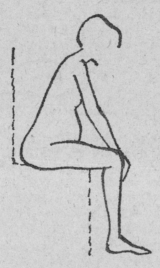

Diagram 22
Backache labour: position 1

head on to your forearms. You will notice that the rules concerning the support of the uterus are again in operation and that you can breathe easily during contractions. In this position you can even read a book propped up in front of you between the contractions.

Position 3. Sit in bed, as for transition stage, but during contractions lean forward and rest your arms on your legs, with the elbows supported on your knees.

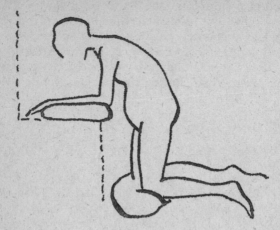

Diagram 23
Backache labour: position 2

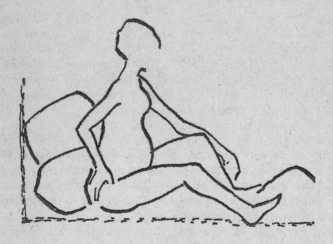

Diagram 24A
Backache labour: position 3

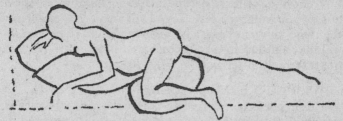

Diagram 24B. Backache labour: position 4

Position 4. This is the same as the alternative lying-down position for transition-stage.

You will usually find that most of the acute discomfort in your back will have disappeared by the time you reach transition-stage. This can be handled in the same way as for ordinary labour; the second or expulsive stage generally follows the normal pattern too. So this backache drill is mainly for handling the first stage of labour.

THIGH-ACHE

This is fairly common although not every woman experiences it. It is thought to be due to the fact that the circulation of blood from the legs to the heart becomes sluggish, because all the pressure in the pelvic area is in the opposite direction. Thigh-ache usually happens towards the end of the first stage of labour but it can be disposed of quite easily. If you feel it, this is what to do:

Sit up as for transition stage or lie on your back, but plant your feet flat on the mattress so that your knees are higher than your trunk. This in itself will provide some relief. If you have your husband with you, ask him to use the palms of both hands to massage firmly upwards from knees to trunk, running them lightly back to the knees again. He should repeat this rhythmically to the end of the contraction.

It may have to be continued for several contractions, but the relief begins immediately.

You can do effleurage while he is using this thigh massage just as you find necessary. If you are alone, you can apply the same kind of massage *between* contractions instead. It will take a little longer to become completely effective, but this is the only difference.

SHIVERING DURING LABOUR

This happens quite often and there are many theories as to why. But what *you* need to know is what to do about it.

You will find that if it happens during your labour, although your teeth may chatter and you may have goose pimples on your skin, nevertheless you will not feel particularly cold. However, extra warmth does provide some relief. A cardigan slipped on or an extra blanket on your bed are very comforting.

In addition, do this between contractions:

Take a deep breath in, hold it to the count of FIVE and then release it as slowly as you can. Repeat this breathing several times if you need to. Possibly you will only manage one of these "holding breaths" between each contraction; but the shivering will only last a little while.

NAUSEA DURING LABOUR

This is not a deviation from normal labour. But it does have unnecessary nuisance-value because it is rather difficult to breathe with control while you are vomiting! It is worth mentioning that I have noticed that women who observe the rule about eating at the *beginning* of the phase of dilatation and *not* eating after that, only suffer very rarely from nausea!

LONG-DRAWN-OUT LABOUR

This certainly seems to happen once in a while and obviously has as its main disadvantage the fact that one does get tired. Often the uterus seems to be working at top-pressure with long, strong contractions and yet the progress of dilatation is slow by comparison.

You will, however, notice, even during a labour like this, that there are periods when the uterus is less active. These periods can be used to take light, easily digestible food (but not milk). You will probably also be offered rather more sedation during such periods; this you should accept, so that you can sleep for intervals and even through the contractions, and awake refreshed for your continued controlled activity. It should by now be very clear that a maximum of sleep is most important during the early pre-labour phase, so that you don't carry a backlog of tiredness with you into the first stage of labour.

The whole of Lesson 7 of course sounds very gloomy because all the difficulties and pain-situations are grouped together. I can only repeat that many women don't experience any of this. Many don't even need effleurage. In fact there are some who don't even need to breathe in Level D and some who don't experience a transition-stage.

If you *have* had a baby before, don't fix your previous experience in your mind as the inevitable pattern of labour for you. Each labour for each woman is different. All the "tools" which I have given you should be ready and available for use in any situation where they may be needed. But don't use any particular breathing-level unless it reaches the point when you *must* in order to maintain comfort. Don t use massage unless you really need it. Decide to handle your labour as it comes and apply the "tools" best suited to it in the actual situation.

It is most essential that all the things I have talked about in relationship to handling labour are *so well rehearsed that they are all semi-automatic*. You should not go into labour trying to remember what the book said, but fully confident that you have made the contents of the book your own equipment.

Lastly, you have to learn what is perhaps the most pleasant "tool" in a normal labour. There will come a magic moment during the second stage of labour when you have been pushing hard for a number of contractions, with the baby's head advancing beautifully all the time. Suddenly the midwife or doctor will say: "With the next contraction I shall tell you to stop pushing and to pant, because the baby's head will be born." This next contraction should be handled gently and *without* the force of your tummy muscles behind it. However, the pushing urge will still be very strong. But you cannot just stop pushing. So you must do something which will mechanically prevent you from making pushing-efforts. For the exact procedure turn to Labour Diagram (6) pages 176, 177.

NOTES ON DELIVERY POSITION

Some midwives like to deliver the baby with the mother lying on her left side. If your midwife prefers this position, ask to be allowed to push on your back until the crown of the baby's head appears. You will find that she will consent to this. But you should understand how she wants you to lie during the baby's birth, so that you can help yourself into this position.

Pull your top-pillow down to waist-level on your *left* side and put your head on the pillow. Next shift your buttocks down until you are lying diagonally across the bed with your head well tucked down and your under-arm pulled forward in front of your chest. Try to look like a crescent. Then bend your right leg and support the knee from underneath with your hand (cup the knee in your palm). With your right hand pull on your right leg as you did when you were making pushing-efforts on your back. Usually your husband, a student, or a pupil midwife will be there to support this leg; but you will still need to pull with your right hand. See Diagram 25.

If your midwife prefers you to stay on your back for the delivery of your baby, you simply lie back against your pillows with your head and shoulders when she says "Stop pushing" then breathe as in Labour Diagram (6).

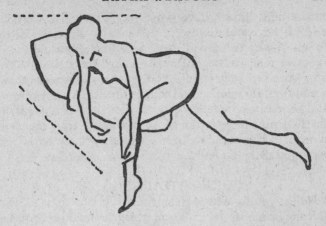

Diagram 25

During the last weeks of your pregnancy ask your midwife or the hospital which position they usually use. *Then practise* Labour Diagram (6) in that position.

You will find that the delivery of the baby's head takes about 10-15 seconds. Then a moment or two later the baby's shoulders will be born. At this point you must obey instructions *instantly*. You may be asked to give "a gentle push" with the next contraction—and they do mean *gentle*. Or you may be asked for "panting" or a combination of the two as required. No one can know this in advance and only the person in charge of the delivery of your baby can judge accurately what is required. After the baby's shoulders have emerged from your body, the rest of his body will slide out. Then your work is done, except for a little assistance with the delivery of the placenta.

And now my work is almost done too. You have all the tools you need. All that remains is for you to rehearse conscientiously until B-Day arrives.

Go over all the lessons again, to make sure that you understand exactly what will be required of you. Check the list the midwife will have given you if your baby is to be born at home and make sure that you have to hand all the things which are needed. You will find a general list of things to take to hospital at the end of this lesson; but do make sure that your hospital does not ask for special things in addition. If it does, add them to the list I have given you. And get everything ready *now*. The pre-labour phase is not the right time to go to the shops for labour equipment any more than it is the time to begin learning exercises. Relax and enjoy these last few weeks.

YOUR HOSPITAL LUGGAGE

Unless you have been given specific instructions on what to bring into hospital with you, this list should take care of your needs:

3 cotton nighties or *3 pairs of cotton pyjamas*. They should be cotton because nylon is too hot to wear in a hospital which will have a higher temperature than your home.

3 bras These should be the last size you wore before you went into hospital or three "Mava" bras which can be used during pregnancy and breast feeding (see index)

3 dozen maternity sanitary towels (size 3)

1 sanitary belt

1 tube Massé cream (for your nipples)

1 cardigan or *bed-jacket*

1 pair of warm socks (husband's will do!)

Your own toilet things: soap, talc, toothbrush etc., make-up, hair-spray, and rollers to pin your hair up, if you generally use them. A mirror which is somewhat larger than the usual powder-compact size will be very useful. Don't forget your deodorant and a bottle of cologne for luxury.

Showercap

1 large box of paper tissues Cotton hankies get crumpled and lost

1 toilet roll Get soft paper like Andrex; hospital-issue is very harsh and uncomfortable after labour.

Books Get several, either from the public-library or from a book-shop. Light fiction will be more readable than a heavy classic but don't rely on magazines—they make a diet which becomes dull very quickly.

Fruit Apples, oranges and bananas. (Not soft fruit, which is best brought by your visitors and eaten while still fresh)

Fruit-squash

Baby-clothes and towels are usually supplied by the hospital during your stay there. But you will need baby clothes later, for when you go home.

Travel to hospital in your dressing-gown and a pair of light shoes. Shoes which have backs as well as small heels are much the most comfortable. Bedroom slippers are *not* the best thing to wear: they usually need to be held on with the toes and this will affect your ease of walking and your posture on those highly polished hospital floors. Your outdoor-clothes are best left at home. Most hospitals cannot usually find the space for them!

LABOUR DIAGRAM 6
SECOND STAGE OF LABOUR: II—Actual birth begins; stop pushing: panting breaths in deep Level C. Be prepared to alternate 'push' and 'don't push' patterns when told to do so.

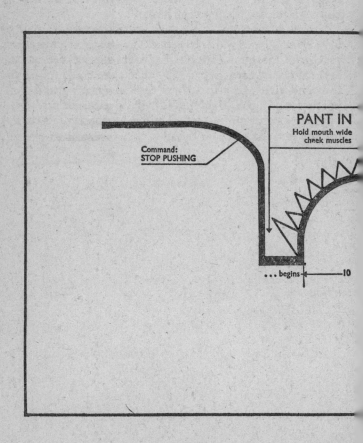

Command:
STOP PUSHING

PANT IN
Hold mouth wide
cheek muscles

... begins

10

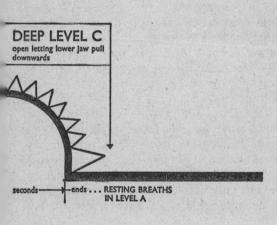

DEEP LEVEL C
open letting lower jaw pull
downwards

seconds —— ends ... RESTING BREATHS
IN LEVEL A

HOME AND DRY—OR IS IT?

WHEN you first realised that you were going to have a baby, perhaps the thought that you would one day have to take care of another human being was not the first thing to occur to you. Many women don't even think about this until after the baby is actually born. For most women there seems to be a neat, pastel-coloured Venetian blind over this aspect of motherhood and it is rudely opened when they come home from hospital with the baby all to themselves for the very first time.

You, however, have prepared for everything. You have taken an active interest in your own health and wellbeing during pregnancy. You have patiently prepared yourself for your role during your baby's birth. So it would be stupid to leave the blind closed over the what, when and why of looking after your baby.

First of all I want to talk frankly about the things you need to buy for baby. You will be at the mercy of shop-assistants who will take your money indifferently for articles which in practice are useless and unnecessary. Mothers, mothers-in-law and grannies will try to persuade you to buy things which in the light of modern knowledge on baby-care are not only unnecessary but indeed undesirable, all because such things were a "must" when you and I were babies.

My mother would be horrified if she knew that I hadn't wrapped my babies in tight swaddling-clothes for the first six months of their independent life. "However did they manage to develop straight arms and legs?" she would say. Well, they did. And they were comfortable into the bargain.

The list of baby-equipment "horrors" is a very long one. But we don't need to examine each item in detail. We only need to look at what is useful and practical *now*.

A simple and perfectly adequate layette would consist of the following items:

3 cellular vests. Look for the kind which are shaped like a T-shirt but with a special "envelope-flap" neckline. (The manufacturers are Chilprufe and Ladybird). These are much better than the classic baby-vests with little ribbons—which becomes knotted and difficult to deal with.

4 Babygrow suits. These serve as both night and dayclothing for the first four to five months. They are available in most baby-shops in pastel colours and are wonderful to use. The baby's body is kept at an even temperature and even when he kicks his covers off he is adequately protected. It is not particularly desirable to have nighties and short day dresses because the change-over means a change in body-temperature.

4 cardigans. These are really only needed for a winter baby who actually needs a cardigan on top of his suit for indoor-wear. No lacy patterns please! They are a snare for small fingers.

3 pairs of mittens. Again for a winter baby only.

3 sleeping-bags. For a winter baby again, these are really invaluable. They serve as outdoor clothing and also as extra nightwear on top of the "Babygrow" suit. They too ensure that baby need never get cold, however active he is while you are sleeping.

3 dozen Turkish towelling nappies. Muslin nappies went out with nursery-maids. Disposable nappies are excellent for travelling, visiting and holidays. But they are usually inadequate after the first six months.

4 pairs water-repellent Marathon nappies. These serve as extra lining inside the towelling nappy. They protect baby's delicate skin against the harmful effects of wetness. They can be washed with the ordinary nappies, but they will dry much faster.

4 pairs plastic pants. Any kind which has proper ventilation such as Playtex or Golden Babe is good. The youngest baby can wear them safely –and your visitors who are "special" enough to be allowed to cuddle your baby will be grateful, too!

Safety-pins. The real nursery ones with special safety catches are safest, but the catch may be somewhat awkward for you to handle. If you like to take a little trouble and sew about 1½ inches of Velcro self-adhesive fabric on to the corners of your nappies (once you have learnt the most convenient way of putting them on of course) then you will find life much easier.

Booties, bonnets, binders, headshawls, lacy knitted dresses and everything with ribbons or tapes—these all belong in a museum.

Now for the larger items:

3 pram-blankets. These should be enough for a summer baby, although you may not use them all by any means if the weather is fine. For the winter you may need two more. These blankets are the small ones which fit a carrycot or pram. The larger cot-blankets can be bought later when you need them for a real cot.

Shawls really are *out*. Their lacy patterns will be a nuisance to you and your baby's fingers will become entangled in them. The weight of a large hand-knitted shawl is also more than any baby should put up with.

4 pairs of cot-sheets. Flannelette or cotton are almost equally good. Flannelette are a little cosier in winter. Babies don't need a topsheet. A very new baby feels more comfortable when it is snugly wrapped, and a carry-cot sheet is an ideal wrapper. The baby needs this only for the first few weeks until he has grown a little more secure in the new large environment which is so different from his snug, small intra-uterine nursery. He will undo his wrappings very firmly when he does not need them any more.

Carry-cot or detachable pram or crib. Any of these will serve him very well as a bed for the first few months. *Don't* put a young baby into a big cot. Would you like to sleep on Exmoor all by yourself? When he grows too long for his carry-cot he can then go into a bigger cot.

Baby bath. There are many baby-baths available with and without stands. Most are either expensive or unpractical. The collapsible sort which fits over your bath is a bright idea—but you will get a backache using it. A large rigid plastic bowl will do beautifully for the first three months. After that the big bath makes a wonderful swimming-pool and it is easy to use if you *kneel* on the bath-mat.

Toiletries. Get a simple cane shopping-basket with a handle which fits over your arm. Line it with plastic or a pretty, washable non-iron material if you wish. This basket should hold the following items:

Baby-powder, nursery-safety pins, cotton-wool in a small container, a baby's hairbrush and small comb, a small pair of blunt-ended scissors, a tube of Morhusept cream.

Do avoid cotton-wool buds on orange-sticks, or any greasy nappy-rash cream if you are using water-repellent liners for your nappies. Oil is usually unnecessary too.

2 large bath-towels. These should be kept for baby's own use.

1 cotton apron with plastic-lining. This is for you to wear while bathing or feeding the baby. Otherwise the pretty new clothes you can now wear will suffer. Many such aprons now have towelling on the outside and plastic on the inside.

Ekco Baby-Sit-ta. This is the present that should be given to every mother by someone who loves her and her baby. You can see it in the baby departments of almost any large store. It will serve as baby's home in the daytime while you are busy with housework. It can be carried in one hand with baby safely strapped into it; it will hang as a car-seat too, and when the baby can sit up but needs support it becomes the first low baby-chair.

The Pram. Shops cash in on your natural pride in your baby. The expensive, high, over-sized pram is a status-symbol perhaps, but is mostly a nuisance which takes up too much space. The type of pram which has a detachable body and folding wheels that will fit into the boot of a car will take up much less space, is cheaper, and much more useful. A sun-canopy is a *must*. Otherwise baby will suffer inside the enclosed hood if the sun is shining and the weather hot. If you want to leave the pram in the garden or outside shops, you should buy a combined cat-insect net which will cost only a few shillings—and save you much worry.

Mattress. Carry-cots and most prams need an additional mattress. There are several on the market which fit either and are made of rubberised hair. They are cheap and look pretty in their washable, gaily-patterned, plastic covers. If the mattress is covered with waterproof material you don't need additional waterproof cot-sheets.

WARNING: NO PILLOWS. Although there are such pretty non-iron pillowslips in the shops which even have "baby" embroidered in one corner, pillows for babies are both unnecessary and dangerous. When the baby is old enough to sit up in his pram he can have a pillow tucked behind his back for comfort. But it should be taken away whenever he lies down. If you can avoid using a pillow in his cot or bed until he is old enough to ask for one, all the better. My own children didn't ask for pillows until they were old enough to sit up in bed to read before getting-up time. The spine and back muscles grow more strong for being allowed to function correctly. The exception to this rule is if a doctor specially requests that the child's body be raised above the waist during certain illnesses.

Bottles. Even if you intend to breast-feed, have a baby's bottle and two teats with medium-sized holes available. If you have to leave the baby while you are away for a few hours, an emergency meals service for him is very useful. A tin of SMA dried milk will make a good emergency supply.

Dummies. Fashions concerning dummies change as fast as do fashions in hem-lines. The latest trend is to say that if baby sucks his fingers pretty often, he is indicating a need to suck which is not completely satisfied while he is on the breast or taking his bottle. In such a case a dummy is better than his fingers, because it is softer and less likely to distort the shape of the gum. The habit will naturally lessen as a child grows up and develops widening interests.

Potties. Don't, don't . . . *please* don't buy one! Read the section on page 192 of this chapter about toilet-training!

Looking after baby-things. When you have bought your baby-clothes and nappies, there is no need to wash anything which was sold in a closed plastic bag before baby wears it. Garment and nappies which were taken out of open plastic envelopes or off the shelf in the shop should be washed before wear. *Never* use detergent on any baby clothes. Use a good, bland soap, Lux Soap flakes or Boots' Babyflakes. If your local water is exceptionally hard, Calgon water softener will remedy this.

Take all the baby's things out of their individual bags and put clothes and nappies away into drawers. Then cover them with plastic sheets to protect them against dirt. This is easier than having individual bags when the clothes are actually in use.

Wash the new pram and carry-cot and any other similar items in warm water with mild detergent added: this removes dust and will satisfy you that neither colour nor paint is likely to come off.

When you return from hospital, or when the midwife has made her last visit, it will be up to you to arrange a daily routine which suits both your household and your baby—and which allows you a little time to be YOU! I know this sounds almost impossible. All your friends will have told you that a baby is a full-time job. But actually it need not be quite that bad if you realise that your baby is not a strange new species but a human being, who therefore has similar needs to yours and mine. These needs are basically food, rest, stimulus, protection, and—most important of all—his parents' love. So let us look at these needs in detail.

FOOD

The baby under twelve weeks old will usually need only milk as both food and drink. Breast-feeding is a much discussed subject, and you will have been inundated with advice about it. It is true that breastmilk is cheaper than any other, that it usually suits the baby well and that it is always available at the right temperature. BUT—and it is a big "but"—none of these facts mean a thing if you hate the idea of feeding your baby from the breast or if your body does not produce the right amount of milk easily. A *struggle* to feed one's baby at the breast, if it is a struggle, is much more upsetting to the baby than serene meal-times with a bottle.

There is one factor which is hardly ever mentioned in connection with breast-feeding yet it seems odd that it isn't, for it is the most important factor connected with feeding a young baby. The baby has lived for 40 weeks in the closest possible proximity with its mother's body. Now, having begun to live independently, it misses this close physical contact. Breast-feeding mechanically ensures that the baby has this contact with its mother's body at regular intervals each day. One cannot feed a baby on the breast and hold it at a distance.

However, one can feed a baby with a bottle and still cuddle it closely while doing so. One woman I knew who could not breast-feed her baby always undid her bra while bottle feeding her baby so that he would feel close to her body and could make direct contact with her skin. This was lovely to see and particularly suited her. But ordinary close cuddling suits most women and their babies very well under circumstances when breast-feeding is for some reason not possible.

A kind of rule can be stated on this:

What you feed to your baby is secondary to
how you do it.

Having said this, let us think about *breast-feeding* more objectively. Hospitals must have a strict routine on feeding times; the number of mothers and babies they care for would make a more permissive routine impossible. But when you get home, do realise that you baby will be hungry, not when the clock says he should be, but when his stomach says. Do *you* eat at precisely the same times every day if you have the choice? Allow your baby the privilege to eat when he wants to as well.

Experienced mothers have a rule: "Never wake a sleeping baby—he'll wake soon enough by himself." Sometimes he will sleep for six hours between feeds; but at other times he will wake and cry after only three hours. So you will adapt to his needs. And soon this will accommodate you too because the baby will show you his individual pattern of needs and you can then build your own routine round it. This does of course include feeding in the "wee small hours" if your baby asks for it.

Often a baby is not actually hungry during the night but just needs the reassurance of your presence. He needs to feel close to you and a small snack is comforting at the same time. Surely you sometimes wake up in the middle of the night feeling a bit unsettled and it occurs to you that a cuppa would not come amiss? Your baby simply needs this more often during his early weeks of living independently. I am assuming for purposes of this book that your breast-feeding has been organised and established by the midwives before you get home. In the index at the end of this book you will find details of a good little leaflet on breast-feeding which can be obtained by writing for it. It was written by a midwife who made breast-feeding her special subject.

If you are breast-feeding and want to go out, to a theatre for example, always leave a bottle of made-up milk mixture (see page 182) with the person who is looking after the baby in your absence. This is obviously not necessary if you are just going shopping down the road, but only if you will be away for four hours or longer. But allow for possibilities. You cannot know about every traffic-jam in advance and the thought of your starving baby will not help your peace of mind.

If you must go out to some social function where you know that you will be away for a long time, you may have to retire to the ladies' room and express your milk otherwise you may find that your over-full breasts leak through your bra and its pads and on to your dress. Not every woman is so bountifully supplied, but many are.

Keep your nipples (the areola) supple by using a little Massé-cream on them, in much the same way that you use hand cream on your hands. Do this after each feed. Before baby goes on the breast next time wipe any surplus off with a tissue.

The same general rules concerning times, etc. apply to *bottle-feeding*. But there are different points to watch. The number of branded milks suitable for babies is considerable; you will most likely find that the one your hospital or midwife has selected suits your baby. How can you tell? Your baby will seem contented after feeds, will sleep well, take his food eagerly and gain weight adequately. Consult the health-visitor, who will come to see you a few days after the midwife has left, about what is an adequate weight-gain for your baby.

A further sign that all is well is that the baby's stools are of a soft texture and mustard-ish brown in colour. By the way, for the first few days after birth, the stools of a new baby are black or very dark green in appearance. This is quite normal, so don't worry about it. Also, a breast-fed baby tends to have more stools than a bottle-fed baby.

These stools are golden in colour and often almost like thin cream in consistency, compared with the darker and firmer stools of the bottle-fed baby. Frequency of stools is much less important than consistency.

But to get back to bottle-feeding. Sterilisation of bottles and teats is very important. You can sterilise them by boiling, but it is a hazardous business and many bottles, glass or nylon, either crack or melt. Teats burn only too often.

In the long run it is easier and safer to sterilise with Milton fluid. Each bottle of Milton carries exact instructions on how to do this and it is a process recommended by hospitals. Milton can be bought by special request in the 16 oz. nursing-home size. You can ask your chemist to apply for it directly to the makers. And Tupperware make beautifully bowl-shaped containers with close-fitting lids, which the makers of Milton recommend. Dummies and teats can be sterilised at the same time as bottles.

During his first few weeks of independent life, your baby should be given his bottle by you as often as possible. Feeding-time is getting-to-know-you time. After about a month, encourage those members of the household who will be with you for a long time to occasionally feed the baby too. Father, granny if she is a regular and frequent visitor, perhaps even an *au pair* girl if you are lucky enough to have one with you for several months.

All these people need to be familiar to your baby, if their share in looking after him is to be easy and pleasant for him, as well as make life easier for you. Each time someone feeds a baby with a bottle and the baby is allowed to enjoy this—is spoken to and patted and changed by that person—a happy relationship is fostered. It is unfair for a complete stranger to suddenly thrust a bottle into a three-month old baby's mouth if he has never had this experience. This doesn't mean that you should keep him entirely to yourself until then. Allow him to meet the household. "Meeting" in this sense is not merely a distant head bent over the cot, but personal physical contact. However, you should still remain the person he meets most frequently.

WEANING

The official rule is that weaning can begin when a baby weighs 15 lbs. or reaches three months of age. This is fair enough; but many babies need the addition of a little solid food before then.

If your baby, whether breast or bottle-fed, suddenly seems unsatisfied at feeding-time even though he has been quite contented until then, you can either increase the amount of milk he gets at every feed or try him with a teaspoon of baby ceral, mixed to a thin cream with warm boiled milk and a little glucose and given just before his tea-time feed. Feed him gently with a spoon and then let him have his usual feed. This may do the trick.

He will be satisfied for a few weeks; then you may find that he needs a little cereal before his midmorning feed also. If he rejects this don't despair. Don't force him. Just try again before the next feed. Some babies are very conservative and accept new things only with great caution. Don't you know adults like this? The "baby book" supplied by most clinics, which is also given away by the baby-departments of many large stores, has an excellent and easy-to-follow weaning-chart.

REST

Young babies sleep for longer than children and adults. But most of them don't sleep for 20 hours out of 24 the way the books say. So at night the baby should not have his cot next to your bed. You will each disturb the other. Put the cot at the other end of the room or better still into the baby's own room. If you are afraid that you might not wake up if he cries, a "baby-alarm" is a good investment.

The room where the baby sleeps should be ventilated even at night, but in the winter there should also be some form of all-night background heating in the room. If you take the baby out of his warm bed and change him in an icy room, he may catch cold. Paraffin-stoves are *not* a suitable background-heating. Beware also of gas-heaters for this purpose. Electric convectors and all-night solid fuel burners are the best.

Your baby will not stay happily in his own room all day as well as all night; he will be aware, even a week after his birth, of being shut away from contact with others. Take his crib or cot into the room where you are working, watching T.V., or whatever. He will enjoy hearing everyday noises and in fact fall asleep much more readily.

Music of any kind is the best way I know to get a baby who is disinclined to sleep all relaxed and drowsy. A baby who sleeps quite well in the day-time yet screams as soon as he is expected to sleep in the dark may need a small night-lamp to reassure him.

Sleeping out of doors is healthy and even the youngest baby enjoys it. The only time he should not be out of doors is during fog or if the temperature is below freezing-point. Even if he is well wrapped and his skin is warm, it is still dangerous for him to breathe in freezing air. If you live upstairs in a flat, and don't like to leave your baby down in front of the house where passers-by may disturb him, it is a good tip to have a solid table near a wide open window and leave the cot on this for most of the day. The baby will get just as much air and without being disturbed by well-meaning old ladies. He can also be heard easily if he cries. You must *not* do this of course when he begins to be able to sit up. If he now sleeps in a big cot, take him away from the open window. Babies have been known to undo the catch on a cot and many babies learn to climb earlier than mothers realise.

After the first few weeks, a daily trip to the park or nearest green area will do both of you a lot of good. But "fresh air" should not mean lying in a howling gale or even in a little draught!

STIMULUS

It is not generally realised that young babies under 12 weeks of age need mental stimulus and get bored if they don't get it. The primitive woman who carries her baby wherever she goes does not have any problem with this. Her baby sees and hears all around him all the time and when he gets tired he just sleeps.

However, in our society many babies are fretful. People don't seem to realise that they should not be expected to sleep all the time unless they are actually being fed or bathed. This is just not fair to *any* human being, however young. Let him decide how much sleep he needs. How? The EKCO Baby Sit-ta I mentioned earlier in this lesson will be your answer. You can put the baby into it after his meal and have the Baby Sit-ta on a table in the kitchen or in the living-room.

Baby will be held safely but he can still look around and see everything that's going on. He can see you and you can see him, without stopping your work. (A cot has sides which he can't see through, but the Baby Sit-ta hasn't.)

Watching you at work, being spoken to and listening to noises—this is what he needs. You don't have to speak in whispers because there is a baby in the house. Ordinary noises like taps running or the vacuum-cleaner going and so on are fun to hear. But doors banging are less fun . . .

Most babies have one definite period during each day when they tend to be awake and somewhat less contented than usual. Use this period for activity such as walks, shopping and general play-time. Feed your baby a little earlier after this interval and it will become a time to look forward to rather than dread.

Babies should have a daily bath—but not for hygienic reasons. A bath is relaxing and enjoyable. Do make tea-time the bath-time. A bath uses up a lot of a baby's energy and the meal which *follows* it usually goes to a very hungry small person. Then the next few hours are spent in blissful sleep—while mummy and daddy have a peaceful evening all to themselves.

PROTECTION

This aspect of a baby's needs falls into three categories: temperature, hygiene and health. And this means comfort, too.

TEMPERATURE

Check that your baby is neither too hot or too cold at any time. Slip your hand inside his bedcovers and inside his leggings and feel his thigh. If it is just comfortably warm but not perspiring, all is well. If his thigh is too cold or too hot, adjust the amount of clothing on his cot. In very cold weather the baby will need mittens and possibly a helmet for outdoors but most babies try valiantly to get rid of both. In hot weather a baby may feel thirsty between feeds. His special orange juice diluted with cool water will be very welcome.

Do use some form of vitamin preparation, especially vitamins A and D, during the winter. If your baby will not take cod-liver oil, ask what the Health Visitor would recommend and follow her advice. Make use of the immunisation and vaccination scheme at your local welfare-clinic. You will appreciate the sense of security brought by your knowledge that you have done your best to protect your baby against disease.

HYGIENE

I shall start by discussing the subject over which there is

more argument than about any other aspect of the care of young children!

Toilet-training. Ignore the well-meant but bad advice of all those friends who have a "clean baby" at six months! It is not fair to impose toilet-training on a young baby. I am not speaking of cruelty or force, but something quite different.

To a small baby the act of excretion is pleasurable. He actually enjoys being able to keep the results of his excretion for a little while. And if he has to use a pot he is deprived of this pleasure. At the time all may seem to be well; but years afterwards untold harm may come to light. Many children who are accused of "holding on" to their stools and who as a result become constipated were given toilet-training too early in life. Many others, who become anxious or even frantic when they need to go to the toilet and there is no convenient opportunity, also have a similar early training behind them.

Is this *really* worth it? Mrs. Jones next door is welcome to her "clean" baby. Wouldn't you rather have an emotionally happy child?

When and how to introduce the pot? Produce one at about 15-16 months (with a shield for a little boy!). And produce it as a TOY. It will be very much enjoyed—at first as a hat, a container for bricks, or a kind of quoit. Help him to play with it. Don't use it for its intended purpose at this point but let the bathroom be its "home". Babies are conservative and later the whole business will be easier if the pot already lives there anyway.

After 2-3 weeks of playing with it you can begin to show your baby how to use it properly. Take the baby to the bathroom when you go there. Sit him on the pot while you sit on the toilet. Don't try to explain what you are doing. Just let him sit there. When you leave the bathroom take him with you.

Repeat this new "game" every time you go to the bathroom yourself. After a few days or possibly a week and a half at the most, your baby will suddenly catch on and imitate what you are doing! But do remember, please, to always take his nappy off while he sits on the pot.

Don't exaggerate your praise when he does use the pot; just approve in an ordinary manner. Now introduce whatever word or other term you want to use for going to the toilet. Within a few weeks your child will ask to . . . even if you aren't in the bathroom.

As soon as he does begin to use the pot in this way, discontinue its use as a toy. *Substitute another toy which is new to the child.* Once he is quite able to ask almost every time and to control himself until he reaches his pot, then is the time to begin leaving off his nappies in the day-time and to use pants instead.

Night-training should not start until a child is about 20 months to two years old and certainly not until he is safely dry by day. Put him on his pot before bedtime. Then wake him and try again three hours later and again before *you* go to bed. Be consistent about this! After a while as his control gets better, you need only repeat the pot routine just before you go to bed.

It follows logically that you must be on hand to put him on his pot when he wakes in the morning. After a whole week of having a dry bed each morning put him into pyjamas instead of nappies (with elastic, not tape, in the trousers) and make it possible for him to get out of bed safely to use the pot himself.

You can do this by taking one cot-side off altogether, and getting your husband to cut the legs of the cot down, so that baby sleeps only about 18 inches above the floor. This will first of all make him independent of your help with his toilet activities. It will also teach him to sleep in a bed instead of a cot. Toddlers are not animals who should be kept in cages, and this is what a cot becomes once its safety-value has become outgrown.

Boys take longer to become dry at night than girls. But

however slow your child may be about this, don't fret and don't scold. Toilet-training is not a proof of physical superiority, mental brilliance or any future tendencies. It is nothing to boast about, to feel guilty about, or ashamed about. Most persistent bedwetters outgrow this tendency sooner or later by themselves. Even they form only a minute proportion of the world-population.

Nappies: These days the dreary business of washing and sterilising nappies can be done efficiently in one operation—by using Nappisan. (This is a powder manufactured by the makers of Milton and it is obtainable at any chemists.) You will also need a pail with a close-fitting lid. Add the Nappisan to half a pail of water, as instructed on the box, and just drop the wet nappies into the solution.

Soiled nappies should have loose particles rinsed off before being dropped into the solution. Water-repellent nappies can join the others quite safely.

Once a day take the nappies out of the pail and rinse them in plain cold water without soap or detergent. Two rinses will be adequate. Wring them out, and hang them up to dry. If you cannot hang things out of doors, and hate having a constant line of washing over your head, maybe you can find a coin-laundry nearby. Sixpence in the drying machine will get a whole pail of nappies bone-dry.

Pastel colours must not go into the Nappisan solution or else the colour will bleach out. Cot-sheets can also be washed through successfully in this manner. In other words, apart from blankets, Babygrow suits and the odd cardigan, all of which should be washed in soap-flakes and rinsed carefully, there isn't going to be the huge daily mountain of washing you were dreading. Mothers who are badly organised will let the washing accumulate over a period of days and then it *can* be a nuisance. Well-organised, with-it mothers rinse the nappies through and do the odd little bits of washing once a day—say after lunch. This way it's hardly noticeable and certainly no hardship.

The other aspect of sterilisation of course concerns feeding bottles and teats, which I dealt with when discussing bottle feeding.

A Word About Your Routine

Let house-work go hang if necessary. Concentrate on keeping your baby happy and yourself rested. A mother who is always rushing about never has enough time for baby or husband and wears herself out into the bargain.

Let relatives and neighbours help you. They frequently offer to do bits of shopping but are rebuffed by the new mother's urge to be independent. Be independent later. Use any help which is offered and don't try to prove how tough you are. If you devote your attention to keeping well-rested and healthy (and this includes a sensible diet which still goes easy on those carbohydrates), then you will feel so much more able to enjoy your baby and to give him wholeheartedly the love you have for him and which he deserves.

Please, please remember not to become so immersed in being a mother that you have no time to be your husband's wife. The more you allow your husband to share his child the more he will appreciate you, the more appreciated you yourself will feel and thus the closer will be the bonds between you all.

This is the time to be feminine. All the cologne you have been hoarding since last Christmas should be used now. Let your husband know that you want to be nice *for him.* Don't slop around in an old dressing-gown or wear old slacks and a sweater all the time. Dress as nicely as you can every day, and remember to protect your clothes with your waterproof apron when bathing and feeding the baby.

Deliberately arrange occasions when you and your husband can be alone and enjoy looking especially attractive on these occasions. About a month or so after the baby's birth an outing to a film or a concert will be a well-deserved treat for you both. At this point try to fix some kind of frequent babysitting arrangement with a friend or with neighbours in a similar situation. Then your life can expand once more towards wider horizons.

It is not wrong to have a life along with your husband now that you are also a mother. On the contrary. For your child's sake as well as the happiness of your marriage, this aspect of your life is one of the important things which will be necessary for the successful development of your new family.

THE NECESSARY FATHER

IN my lecture courses on the psychoprophylactic method of childbirth, there is always one evening known as "father's night". At first when I started these, I used to be afraid that no one would turn up—or that only one solitary, frightened man would appear.

But every time I have been gladdened and encouraged to see just how many fathers there are, who are prepared to make an effort to find out what goes on during the birth of their child—and what they can do to help. In fact, the numbers of young men who want to be informed about the contribution they can make are growing overwhelmingly. So in reading this chapter you are taking part in a new and rather surprising cultural trend.

To the best of my knowledge, this growth of interest has never happened before in any society, ancient or modern, eastern or western. Nowhere has there been such an endeavour to have husbands participate *directly* in the birth of their children. There have been, and still are, various ethnic and social groups dotted around this planet in which husbands do participate—but indirectly.

For example, in one West African region there is a very interesting native custom. When a pregnant woman begins to feel what perhaps might be labour, she tells her husband—as all good wives should. This is the signal for him to run. He runs outside his village to a particular bush—not just any old bush but the one which is traditionally the first bush out of earshot. He sits down under this bush, and proceeds to do whatever it is one does do when sitting under a bush. And then his parents take charge of the wife's labour; father-in-law acts as midwife, and mother-in-law as labour companion. (Presumably her job is to say "1-2-1-2

Blow!") Once the baby is safely delivered mother-in-law wraps it in a cloth, carries it to the bush and shows it to the father. This is his signal that all is now safe; off he goes home and much rejoicing takes place.

I suppose this is a kind of participation. It's not just one or two men who feel like running off to this bush; it is the prescribed thing for all men to do so. If on any day in that particular village, there's a rush on, the bush must be somewhat overcrowded. I hardly dare contemplate the possibilities.

But there are other forms of participation which are psychologically interesting from the mother's point of view and, so I gather, valuable as well.

One of these takes place in a part of Mexico still inhabited largely by Indians. Here, when a woman goes into labour she makes her way to a hut outside the village and there she behaves as ritual prescribes that one should in order to give birth to one's child. At the same time, her husband goes to the village square. There he enacts dramatically the suffering his wife ought to have when she is giving birth to her child. And while he is "suffering" he is solicitously attended by the village virgins. (This situation may sound rather familiar to you but unfortunately I don't really think one could seriously advocate such a service in Great Britain today.)

Psychologists tell us that this practice is the reason why this tribe is known to have extremely easy labours. The women are fully reassured by the fact that their husbands are doing the suffering for them. It is obvious that psychologically this *is* perfectly sound—the mothers are taught how to behave sensibly while their husbands do all the suffering. This is one example of Father Participation.

Now although I can't provide the village virgins for you, or the suffering for that matter, I do offer you a service—but a quite different one. The fact that it is completely new in any society doesn't make it any the less valid. What you are being offered is direct active participation of two kinds, and on two levels.

Firstly, participation on a purely practical level. Perhaps the main yard-stick of how a woman should feel in labour is *comfort*. There are many perfectly ordinary, simple services that anyone can render to a woman in labour which will increase her level of comfort; in the course of this chapter I will give you precise instructions on the kind of things to do to make her more comfortable. Of course this is something that is not applicable to you alone. I could do this, and so could any reasonable human being with a little common sense.

But there *is* something more which you can do for your wife—and which no one else can do, neither the obstetricians nor the midwives nor anyone else. And that is *be there*. Because you are *you*, not because you are just another person, but because you are related to your wife by the bonds of marriage. It is this relationship that gives your presence its unique value. It works in two directions of course: after all, the vows of marriage, if you think about them, imply sharing. This is why we get married to a particular person, because we feel (sometimes wrongly) that this is the person with whom we want to share the way we live. And giving birth to a child, adding a new member to the family, is a very important aspect of living. In a way it is *the* most important aspect, particularly at the time when it happens—and far, far more important than a choice of furniture or house or even career. So it ought to be shared as part of a marriage and this is why, if it can be shared, the value to the wife *as a person* is so great and so unique. It isn't merely that she should not be alone; this birth-event should not be a happening completely out of context to the rest of her life. It *becomes* out of context if she cannot, for some reason or other, share all or part of it with her partner.

The value to a wife manifests itself in many different ways. First of all, I am of course assuming, when I say that husband and wife ought to share the birth of their child, that both of them are adequately equipped for the job of having a child. This means, among other things, an understanding of how one conducts oneself during the proceedings which we call labour, and which culminate in the birth of a child. This is only rational; if two people are going for a drive in a car, it is assumed that at least one of them can drive and the other knows at any rate how to sit in the passenger seat! This is a minimum requirement, which no one regards as the least bit odd.

Only in the field of obstetrics do people still think it peculiar that people should want to know what they can do to help when their child is born. This is because the medical profession—and I speak as one of them—has for centuries had a sort of mystique that it doesn't matter about the "owner" of the disease, that he doesn't need to know anything. There's a sort of closed shop on knowledge about bodies and their diseases and what to do with them. Childbirth has in this sense become part of this knowledge, almost a disease about which midwives and doctors have their own mystique. (If any midwives and doctors feel incensed at this, they may by all means send me a rude letter. I don't mind being executed for my opinions—*after* I've had a chance to talk about them.)

So when I talk about the sharing of this experience between two people who are adult enough to have discovered how to share, what I mean in the context of childbirth is: a woman who has trained to understand her contribution to her child's birth and a husband who has trained to understand how best to help her make that contribution. This is really what "The Necessary Father" is all about. I shall teach you, as a husband, to be a sort of plumber's mate to your wife during this job she has to do. (And I choose this description carefully!)

Now—what will be the results? Well, the psychological assistance you render will be invaluable physically, both during labour and during the post-natal period. The fact that one's emotions have a profound effect on one's physiological function is now so well known that we can even dare say it publicly. How a woman *feels* during labour assists her or retards her in terms of her physiological return to normal. The fact that it also strengthens the bond between the partners, almost goes without saying. And from the child's point of view, you are assisting your wife to give it the best possible start in life; the more efficiently she functions physically, the more successfully she handles this happening psychologically and the more efficient her labour will be. Therefore the child's survival reflexes are likely to be in much better condition than those of children born under more orthodox circumstances.

Perhaps I have already convinced you and you are thinking, "Very well, I'll be Sir Galahad! I'll suffer the agonies of being there. I won't be squeamish when I see the blood; I can always look the other way". Well, don't strain yourself. In any case I'm going to offer you a bonus. There will be a great deal in this for *you*. At least, I think so. I can't speak from personal experience, naturally. I know what it's like to give birth to a child, and I know what it's like to have my husband there. However, I have never been anyone's husband! But if the testimony of thousands of trained women is any indication at all, the overwhelming attitude is "I wouldn't have missed it for the world!"

Curiously enough, this is particularly evident among men who the day before were saying "Look dear, don't you think you could really manage without me? I'll come and see you *immediately* afterwards. I don't see honestly that I'd be of any use . . ." Yet even they find themselves caught up in this tremendous experience, for this was the birth of a *human being*—not just a child of theirs. Afterwards they are full of proselytising zeal, and insist this is something everyone should witness. As one husband said, "Why did you try to persuade us? Why didn't you simply issue a life-or-death order: your wife will not survive,unless you're there! How can you just offer a man a choice when you know what is in store for him?"

Why? Obviously because you are human beings and all human beings have the privilege of choice. I and my fellow workers are not yet at the stage when we are willing to dictate that which is good for you. Occasionally there are governments who attempt to do this. But I have noticed that even on the subject of cigarette-smoking, democracy still exists.

But why is this experience so important and beneficial to you? I must admit that I do think that perhaps all human beings, not only husbands, ought to have the opportunity at least once in their lives of witnessing the birth of a child. The experience of watching another human being arrive and become a member, not only of his immediate personal family, but also of the family of *homo sapiens*—this *is* a very profound and deeply moving experience. Whether one sees it once or a thousand times, one can never avoid being involved. Every midwife and every doctor becomes involved anew in this excitement every time. You may not be able to see this of course; and in hospital they're all hidden behind those masks, so you can't see anything. A clipped voice will remark "There you are now, that was splendid. Don't you feel proud?" and the voice will sound, apparently, completely unemotional. But I don't know of any doctors or midwives who don't feel a lump in the throat when they meet each new baby, however many they may have met before.

There is a film on the psychoprophylactic method, which some of you may see in the future, called "Birthday". Now this film was shot by perfectly ordinary cameramen. They were warned beforehand about what they were going to see; although all of them had to be married and fathers of children, none of them had ever seen an actual birth. I prepared them as well as I could by showing them photographs and diagrams; I thought it might be disastrous if one of them fainted while in charge of a camera. The results were, however, rather unexpected. At one point in the film, the mother reached down to grasp her child. As she did so she said "Hello baby!" Recognising that this would make a beautiful shot I had stepped back out of the camera since I wasn't at that moment needed. As I did so, I glanced round and saw that two of the cameramen were openly crying. When I asked them if they were all right the only reply was, "Don't worry—the cameras are turning". But I knew how they felt.

This experience is all the more valuable if this human being whose birth you are witnessing is someone with whom you will spend many years in close and intimate relationship. And further, it gives you a unique opportunity of beginning this relationship *right now*, not several hours later through a pane of glass. "That's yours" is hardly the beginning of a relationship! Nor is ten days later, when your wife brings home the child for the first time. But the moment when she begins her active relationship with the child as a separate human being, and not just something kicking and moving inside her body. And if you *both* begin this relationship together, this is the best effect of all. Many couples soon realise why: *no woman whose husband has been willing and privileged to share this experience with her will ever become possessive about this child.* From the start the baby belongs to them both.

And equally no husband who has participated to this extent can surely ever be quite as unwilling to participate in the child's active upbringing as perhaps your father was. I know that to my father I hardly seemed to exist until the day I brought home my first school report. Then he patted me on the head and gave me a shilling, and that was the beginning of our relationship! To this day my father seems just a strange, shadowy figure who was around. He paid for things; he was someone to get things from, perhaps if my mother refused. Usually he never heard half of what I said to him because he couldn't be bothered to listen, and when he was tired of the story would just say, "Yes all right".

That's not having a relationship. I may be generalising, but I'm pretty sure this happens to many of us. Most people have a much more intimate relationship with their mothers than with their fathers, and this is not just accidental.

And here, perhaps to the regret of some mothers, I am offering you the recipe to end this monopoly. Much as mothers might sometimes think it desirable, this state of affairs is wrong. It's wrong because a child is a member of the whole family and not the "property" of one particular partner. But this question doesn't arise in a situation where both the original partners who founded the child have been able to share the relationship with the child and subsequent children—from the beginning.

We know already that this is so. In other countries where this method of training has been used much more freely and over a much longer period of time, it has been found that the children born by this method adapt themselves in many ways to family and social life much more successfully than others. We also know that women who have successfully dealt with the challenge of giving birth with the great degree of control it is possible to enjoy, can also adapt themselves to the correct role of a parent much more easily.

So this is yet another and perfectly logical benefit: your correct place in this set-up called the family.

But—to achieve all this, it just isn't enough for you to be willing to sit there and merely stick it out. You have to understand what you're doing. You have to know exactly what your wife's doing, why she's doing it, how best to assist her to do it, and what you yourself should be doing to help. This is what this chapter is all about.

You should start by studying—if you haven't already done so—the diagrams on the female reproductive system (page 228 and 231) and the diagrams representing the course of labour (page 92). Look at the process of labour from the purely physiological angle; then you will be able to recognise everything when it happens with your eyes and ears and not by referring to notes.

By all means make notes, but don't do what one husband did with his. He knew that they were important so he put them in a safe place. On "the day" he did everything properly for the first "leg" of his wife's labour, and at the correct moment he called the ambulance. The ambulance arrived promptly, his wife was put in and he was about to follow.

Suddenly he exclaimed "Oh, I've forgotten my labour notes! Just hang on a minute" and off he rushed upstairs. Ten minutes later, he was still searching his belongings when the ambulance driver appeared in the bedroom.

"Look mate", he said, "either you come now or we ain't going nowhere!"

"Why?" he said distractedly, not even looking round.

"Because otherwise we're having it right now, that's why!"

So off he had to go. That was eight months ago—and he hasn't been able to find them since.

Keep your labour notes in some familiar place, such as that old sports jacket you won't let your wife throw away because you always like to wear it when you want to feel comfortable. (Like a woman's handbag your notes really ought to be fastened to your wrist with a chain!)

WHY MAN'S WORK IS NEVER DONE

LIKE any other specialised activity, birth has its own peculiar jargon. You will have to get used to this in order to "translate" it to yourself.

Midwives and doctors always talk about birth in "stages". They will say "She"—she being the woman concerned—"is doing such-and-such." Actually they don't mean this at all. What they do mean is that the body of her uterus is doing this, that, or the other to her cervix. So they say, "She's first staging nicely". In other words, the first stage of labour is well in progress with this particular patient. Or "She's dilating nicely" is a phrase you may frequently hear. This is because when we refer to the opening of the cervix, we use the Latin term *dilatation*. And in England we measure the amount of the opening with fingers. Therefore we talk about it, in England, in terms of fingers! Everywhere else in the Western world they refer to it in centimetres.

Once upon a time everyone used to refer to it in terms of coinage, the coinage of the particular country concerned. So in England we talked about a "sixpenny dilatation" or a "threepenny dilatation" (you know, that tiny silver coin we used to have) or a half-crown dilatation or a crown (or five shillings) dilatation. The French did the same with their coinage and the Russians, and the Chinese too.

Now there were two things about this which made life rather difficult. One was the fact that the coins of the realm change now and then. I mean, no modern midwife in this country would know what a five-shilling dilatation was! She would probably never have seen an old crown piece. Secondly, after World War II international conferences became fashionable. And every year obstetricians from all over the world, like many other bodies, got together to argue with obstetricians from other countries instead of merely with those from their own. They soon realised that to talk about "what you do when she's two yen dilated" isn't the same thing at all as "what you do when she's half-a-rouble dilated"; the British obstetricians with their half-crowns and five-shilling pieces were just not considered, and it was mutually agreed by everybody else to do the measuring in centimetres. The poor British—driving on the left, and measuring in fingers!

But in fact this system isn't unreasonable, because the measuring is actually done with fingers. The doctor or midwife establishes the degree of dilatation objectively by passing two fingers into the vagina and feeling how much of those two fingers they can get into the cervix, the opening at the top of the vagina. At first the cervix is tightly closed; then it gradually begins to open; the midwife examines and says "Hm, two fingers" and so on. Eventually some hours later "Ah—I could drive a bus round here—she's half-dilated now!" And finally, she'll be fully dilated. So when you hear these terms you will know what they mean.

DON'T please, follow the example of the husband who rang me up to tell me his wife was two fingers dilated. I asked if the midwife was there. No. Had she been? No. "Then how do you know," said I, "that she's two fingers dilated?" "I examined her" said he.

I managed to put down the telephone before I fainted! He was deadly accurate, but that wasn't the reason. Never, never do this examination yourself. You run the risk of seriously infecting both mother and baby if you do. There are fairly accurate subjective means of establishing the course of labour without using your fingers!

Before labour proper begins (and the phase of dilatation is labelled the first stage of labour) a thinning or shortening of the muscles of the cervix has to take place. This is a "pre-labour phase". For about 30% of women it takes place without anyone being any the wiser. During the last week or ten days of pregnancy, your wife will tell you about "testing contractions". "Feel this!" she will proudly say. These contractions perform the physiological function of very gently shortening and thinning the cervix. If this has been happening you will only know when suddenly the much stronger dilatation-phase contractions apparently start to happen out of the blue! You will have forgotten that she has been saying "feel this" for the last week or so.

Actually there's no guarantee about this. Quite often a woman gets the same strength of contraction during that last week or so; yet before labour proper, the phase of dilatation, begins, she will have a pre-labour phase of various combined and characteristic symptoms lasting several hours. You just can't tell.

Obstetrics is altogether a very chancy business. There are so many unknown factors that no-one can tell you about, but which you discover quite easily at the time. The only thing you must not do is get the idea fixed in your mind that "It's going to be like so-and-so". You must be especially careful if you have been through this game before. "It's going to be the way it was before" is just so much rubbish. There is absolutely no guarantee that it will be like anything. The variability of factors is so very great.

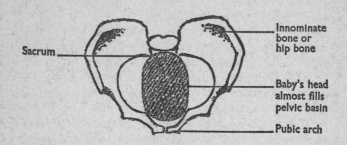

Diagram 26A
The Pelvis at end of Pregnancy

If the thinning of the cervix does take place as a pre-labour phase, you should look out for the following things:

(a) *Short, weak contractions:* Now how are you to know whether they are weak, medium-strong or strong? Well, if your wife has done her training properly she will be breathing properly—and this is how you will know.

If she is still handling her contractions easily with Level A breathing—in other words still working on the Labour Diagram (1) contraction pattern—then they are weak contractions. And if they are no longer than 45 seconds (not minutes!) each, then they are short contractions.

If your wife is booked in at a hospital, they will probably have already given you one of those pamphlets which says: When the pains (they mean contractions) come every 10 minutes, go to your hospital. Let me tell you right now that the intervals between contractions don't mean a thing. In 1894 people thought they did and the booklet has not yet been revised. The only phase which *is* important, as a means to diagnose what's happening, is that during which the uterus is *in action*. Not when it is at rest. So use the length and strength of the function bit, i.e. the contraction, and *not* the intervals between, as your guide as to whether you should telephone yet.

This is of course the thing that everyone wants to know—"When do I phone?" I'll tell you later on when you *do* phone; but for now, the strength and length—with anything up to 45 seconds in length—will tell you if the cervix is still thinning. All you do at this stage is stay at home, preferably in your bed.

(b) *Specific emotional changes:* You will unfortunately be the victim of these—as you usually are in other situations too!

First of all comes a tremendous boost of energy. This of course is to prepare the body for the hard work ahead. But it happens somewhat in advance.

14

Next there is an unmistakable but very pleasant excitement. It's like the feeling you get the day before you go on holiday: you may be terribly busy and active with passports and currency and odd jobs, but in your solar plexus you have a kind of giddy, bubbly feeling. A woman has exactly the same feeling accompanying the phase of thinning of the cervix. If she gets it as a special phase you will be directly affected—because what goes with it is an irresistible urge to tell someone. If this begins in the daytime, wives usually phone their husbands. Some even phone me if their husbands travel around on the job and they know they can't get hold of them. Sometimes they use some pretext or other, such as losing their post-natal leaflet. Knowing this, I ask if they are due to come to a class. Then they say almost casually, "Well no; I think I'm starting in labour". But if this begins at night, as it so often does, they have a victim lying ready to hand, sleeping the sleep of the just . . .

The following instructions, then, are for your benefit, too. When this happens, she will really be waking you much too early. But this is an enormous burst of nervous energy—one feels one could take the tiles off the roof and put them all back again. And because the urge is so strong, you can't really tell a woman that it's quite unnecessary to wake you up and what she should do is just turn over and go to sleep again! Emotionally she just *can't*.

So we combine two things: we use up some of the energy and make life a little easier for you. Her instructions are: She gets up quietly, without waking you. She goes and spends a penny—all pregnant women who get up in the middle of the night *have* to go and spend a penny, for physiological reasons which are obvious if you look at the contents of the pelvis. Then she makes two cups of whatever is an acceptable drink in your house at half past two in the morning.

Please don't be bamboozled into getting up and making the drink for her yourself. She's not an invalid. It is *good* for her to go and make two cups of something. She is using up some of her surplus energy, and at the same time it does at least take the sting out of it for you, if you have to be wakened up, to be wakened with a nice cup of something!

As soon as she *does* wake you up, your job begins. She will be having a few contractions, irregular still and quite weak. The whole trick is to get her into a harmonious working relationship with her uterus NOW— not when it is practically slapping her in the face, which is somewhat late. It should start at the beginning—at Labour Diagram (1).

So watch for it. Perhaps she'll be sitting by your bed with a cup of tomato soup; and suddenly she says "Oh—I've got a contraction." At this point you should say "Right, put your cup down and breathe." Do it right now. Not later. And continue from now onwards, with every contraction while she's awake in the normal course of things.

She doesn't have to lie down supported by pillows in various directions; sitting in a chair, with her body completely relaxed and breathing in Level A, is perfectly adequate. When the contraction has gone, some 35 seconds later, she can pick up her cup and carry on drinking.

When she's finished her drink, please discourage her from spending the rest of the night bouncing about. Of course it's very tempting; emotionally one wants to. And you know how women are terribly good at finding themselves lots of little jobs to do! At this stage of labour there shouldn't be any "little jobs" to do. She should have packed her suitcase earlier, but even if she hasn't it can wait. If she is having the baby at home and you haven't got the jug, the jam jar and the newspaper ready, then tomorrow morning will do. So back to bed—and it's almost a case of *must;* otherwise, if she spends the rest of the night bouncing around and the pattern has to try and establish itself all through the next day, then by the time she gets into labour, her body will not be fit to handle it. Just get her back into bed, whatever you do. Let her read for half an hour perhaps, so that her nervous system can settle; then if necessary hit her on the head with a rolling pin. But if you remind her of the original decontraction drill she learnt, this will help her to go to sleep more easily.

By the morning (or at least when it's time to get up) she may still not have advanced any further, especially if it's a first baby. Just these weak odd contractions and nothing much else. Even if you're going to be with her during labour, you should go to work.

DO NOT sit at home, stop-watch in hand, counting every contraction. The pattern at this stage is very delicate and the slightest thing can make it stop. If you sit there, as many conscientious husbands have done before, saying "Darling, do you know it's six-and-a-half minutes since the last one", the midwife will still be popping round next Christmas to see how you're getting on.

You can go off—but your wife should be able to reach you whenever she wants to. Make it possible for her to know where you are if you're likely to be in an office.

This situation may continue for two or three days—or only for three hours. Characteristically it is handled by trained women in this way:

(1) Normal everyday housework; extra rest in between; more rest afterwards. In other words this is the day on which she should take, even if she hasn't done so for the whole previous nine months, that famous afternoon sleep for pregnant women. If you are a sensible husband, you will ring her up at half past one to make sure what she's doing. And even if you wake her up, at least you will know that she was doing her bit!

You see, women get this nervous excitement and forget all these things. So your job is to be the steadying influence, to remind her that she is supposed to lie down for the afternoon. She may only lie there without going to sleep, perhaps listening to Woman's Hour on the radio. But I've never heard of any woman yet (who wasn't in established labour) who didn't feel sleepy by the time it was over!

(2) In the evening: Supper, bath and bed before 10 p.m. If she can't sleep—and this is fairly common—she can watch television as long as her body is resting, or she can read.

Gradually, whether it is a matter of hours or days, this pattern will change. It changes as follows:

First, two symptoms may occur. On the other hand they may not until much later, but you must know about them, otherwise you won't know what to do. The first one is called a "show". You can see from Diagram 18 the plug of mucus in the cervix. This plug will gradually come out during the course of the first stage of labour. It appears as a slightly blood-stained mucus discharge. To qualify "slightly blood-stained" I don't mean bright red blood by the half-pint. It should be a mucus discharge, slightly blood-stained.

Your wife won't feel this; she will just suddenly announce "I've had a show". Splendid. You should have a piece of paper by the telephone (that's where you're going to need it). On it you write SHOW AT 2.30 P.M. or whenever it was.

The second thing is this: The baby inside the uterus floats in a water-filled bag of membrane. This looks very much like a polythene bag full of water.

Now, this bag may spring a leak. And I am speaking literally! Many women when they first experience this sensation think "As if I haven't enough to think about—now I've lost control of my bladder!" They haven't of course, but it feels suspiciously like it.

If this happens, write on the piece of paper: MEMBRANES LEAKING AT... You will need this information, too, when you phone the midwife or the hospital.

Alternatively, the leak may repeat several times during the next few contractions, or the bag of membranes may burst. The difference between the two will be immediately obvious from the quantity of liquid. If the bag of membranes does burst or trickle any time before you actually reach the hospital (if that's where you're going), phone the hospital immediately to tell them. If it's merely trickling you can tell them later—when you'll be telling them lots of other things as well.

If it's a home confinement, phone the midwife and say clearly "Mrs. So-and-So has been having weak contractions since . . . and the bag of membranes has just burst". This is important, because in this case the baby is now open to infection, and midwives like the mother to be where she can have an eye kept on her.

When the midwife comes, she will examine her and then decide what to do. Usually she merely says she ought to go to bed; obviously she doesn't want her rooting about in the coal cellar in that state. So if the bag of membranes bursts, at this point you drop everything and phone the hospital. But if it's only leaking slightly, you don't.

Again, none of this may happen until much later, in which case you don't have to phone anyone. But the one change that *will* take place is this: gradually the contractions become stronger. How will you find out? Because you have ears—and you will have been accustomed to hearing the constant steady, slow, "Breathe-in-blow!" with every contraction, and to measuring the length of the contraction from the very first intake of breath to the very last blow.

Suddenly you'll hear the steady breathing in and blowing out—and then you'll hear it change to Level B breathing and become slightly quicker. Then it will slow down again. And you will notice that the contraction is some 52 seconds long. It has become longer and she's now breathing in the upper level.

Don't panic—just listen. Listen for half an hour, even if this is her ninth baby. If for half an hour she has been doing Labour Diagram (2) breathing (remember Labour Diagram

(2) is on pages 98-9), and the contractions are 55 to 60 seconds in length from the first breath in to the last breath out, you can safely assume that labour proper—or the phase of dilatation—has begun.

Half an hour of medium-strong Labour Diagram (2) contractions, 55 seconds to one minute long, and this is it!

Then you do the following things:

(1) Assist her to have a bath—in the sense that you remind her to go and have it, not that you stay and scrub her back. You can do that too if you like, but this is not a bath to be clean with. This is a therapeutic bath, as hot as is comfortable and as your hot water system permits. And as deep as your bath and her tummy together will allow! (You've probably discovered that this isn't as easy as it sounds, either.)

The hot water will stimulate circulation of blood to the uterus; also the external pressure of water and the internal pressure of water in the uterus will be balanced. These factors make a bath a very pleasant place in which to learn to adapt to the longer, stronger contractions. So the bath has a dual purpose.

By the way, if this happens in the daytime and she rings you at the office to say that for the last 20 minutes the contractions have been medium-strong, etc., *don't* tell her to have a bath. You should go home first. She should *not* be alone in the house having a bath in labour. Also, the bathroom door must not be locked. Closed yes, but not locked: a woman in labour must never be inaccessible. Equally, she shouldn't be in the lavatory with the door locked.

(2) While she's having her bath—and you'll probably hate this—you should prepare a meal. (By all means let the cook do it if you have one!)

What the meal consists of depends on your taste—and on what time of day it is. If you're going to hospital with her, or if you're going to be with her in labour at home, you should have this meal with her. Even if it is two o'clock in the morning, this meal is an absolute necessity for her. As labour establishes itself, the digestive processes of the body virtually shut up shop; all the available energy is conserved for the uterine function and so less digestion is actually capable of taking place. Later she won't be able to eat but will just be sick.

On the other hand her blood sugar will be used up pretty fast and when she gets to the point when she has to assist the uterus to push the baby out there won't be much left; so we have to find the moment when she can still supplement it safely by eating—and this is the moment! At least it usually is. Once I went to see a woman in hospital who was having rather a long labour. "I can't tell you how glad I am to have got this far" she told me. "Me too," I said. "But what makes you so especially pleased about this moment?" "Well," she replied, "I've just had my fifth last meal."

Hospitals of course are not restaurants. So you're going to get awfully hungry yourself! And your blood sugar is also important so you should eat now too. Curiously enough, husbands who are present for a home confinement should theoretically have a wonderful time in the kitchen. Yet they don't. One is so busy one doesn't seem to have time to even have a sandwich. That's why you should eat now too.

I needn't remind you, naturally, that during this meal whenever she has a contraction she puts down her knife and fork, leans her weight on the table and handles her contraction with breathing.

When the meal is over she may still be at Labour Diagram (2). But it is possible that by this time the contractions are now strong, she has to breathe in Level D at the height of the contraction in order to handle it with control, and its length is just creeping over a minute.

In either case, progress is obviously being maintained. This is the time to notify the powers that be. Telephone the hospital now, if that's where you're going, or the midwife and doctor if the confinement is to be at home. What you tell them is identical, except for one thing! If you phone the hospital, the telephonist on the switchboard will answer you. Don't tell *her* your labour story. All she can do is say thank you and put you through to the maternity ward. Then you'll have to start all over again! Just ask for the maternity ward and sister and you'll be put through. If you're phoning the doctor and midwife, don't forget to give your address in addition to the patient's name.

The following information should then be given to all three:

(i) The length of contraction.
(ii) The strength of contraction.
(iii) Whether there has been a show.
(iv) The state of the bag of membranes—whether it is intact, leaking or just burst, perhaps as your wife got up from the table.

If you have an ambulance card, your next job is to phone for the ambulance. In the Greater London area it takes about 15 minutes from receipt of the call for a maternity ambulance to arrive at the door. Please do tell the ambulance station that this is a maternity patient—then they will be even quicker!

If you are taking your wife to hospital by car, throw a couple of pillows and a rug into the back, if you haven't done so already. In labour it's much more comfortable than sitting in the passenger seat, to lean against a couple of pillows tucked into the back seat, with one's legs up and covered by a blanket.

And if you're driving to the hospital do make sure that you know exactly where it is! You wife may have been visiting the hospital for several months but do *you* know where it is? And what about all those one-way streets? Some time in the last two weeks before the baby is due, take a Sunday afternoon trip to the hospital, just to make sure.

If you're going by ambulance, please ask the ambulance men to put your wife into the ambulance *feet first*. Strange that you should have to do this? All patients going by ambulance, whatever they're going for, go in head first, because feet first has unfortunate connotations! That way, however, one travels with one's back to the engine—and not even passengers on trains like travelling with their backs to the engine. It makes most people feel sick. So feet first for comfort. The ambulance driver may well think you're a little crazy, but then he'll think so anyway when he sees that you're going too—and that you're *not* shivering in your shoes! You should also make sure, of course, that the suitcase is packed before the ambulance arrives. Then away you go.

If the confinement is to take place at home, once you have phoned the midwife and told her all the necessary things, your job is then to make sure that all those things on that famous list are actually available in one place, preferably the room where the baby is to be born. Which list? You know—the one which they give you saying: two jam-jars, plenty of newspaper and so on.

It is quite surprising how many people have the bowl in the bathroom and the bucket in the kitchen and the sheets in the linen-cupboard and the baby's things in the spare room: so the first thing the poor midwife has to do when she arrives is make a grand tour of the house finding all this. It's both irritating and tiring! If you have everything ready in the right room, you will add to her respect for you.

When the midwife comes, or when you get to hospital, the routine is the same. You will be asked to "wait outside" while the first preparations for labour are made. An internal examination is made, her pubic hair is shaved, and various other odd jobs done—all of which will be very boring for you.

There will probably be several other occasions during the remainder of this labour when you will be asked "Please would you mind waiting outside?" So take a tip and take a book. It can be very dull staring at bare walls; it's a good deal less wearing if you have James Bond safely in your pocket and you know that every now and then you can go out, read a couple more pages and then go back again. I remember one man who read through the whole of Goethe during his wife's labour. How he did this, I don't know, but I found him sitting in the corridor completely absorbed and he showed me what it was that was so fascinating. But most people prefer a "who-dun-it".

Then the point will come, either at home or at the hospital, when you are told: "O.K., you can go to her now and she can get on with it."

This is where your real work begins. During the whole of the first stage of labour this work consists of the following things:

During the thinning of the cervix you were encouraging her to sleep as much as possible. But during true labour—the dilatation phase—you should make *every effort* to keep her alert and wide awake. How you do this depends to some extent on what she likes. Some women like being read to. Some prefer to simply sit there and read, with their husband sitting reading next to them. Most hospitals have a radio and if it's daytime she can listen to that; some hospitals even have television.

It is pointless, in fact *dangerous*, to encourage a woman trained to handle her labour with conscious control to sleep between "pains". (This is the word that most midwives use.) The trick is to be as wide awake and alert as possible. So that every contraction is properly handled from its first whisper to its last. So you do your best to keep her entertained.

You should also remind her that she must handle every contraction with the appropriate degree of neuro-muscular control and the appropriate breathing. There is no exception to this rule. She must not continue a conversation or answer questions while she is having a contraction.

Having a contraction is really like being in the middle of prayer—and don't shy away at the term! One doesn't answer questions about when one would like a cup of tea in the middle of prayer; no one would dream of going up and doing this to someone else in church. But curiously enough they will during labour. People constantly come in wanting to know if she is thirsty or comfortable, or to listen to the baby's heart, or because it's Matron's famous daily round.

So if this "Well-mother-and-how-are-we-today?" routine occurs, it is your job to say "I'm so sorry Matron (or Sister or Nurse), but she's in the middle of a contraction". No one has ever caused any offence with this phrase yet. After a while, they get the idea that this woman, for some peculiar reason, is actually *doing* something while she is having a contraction, and so can't answer questions.

Many people are quite convinced that patients in labour are imminently dying of malnutrition; never are they so careful to offer hot drinks, light meals, etc., as in labour. But the digestive system just does not absorb food during established labour, including glucose sweets or barley sugar. Indeed any sugar merely causes people to be sick. If it must be given, the only kind of sugar which can be absorbed is through the circulation intravenously. We've tried all sorts of liquids—fruit juice, tonic water, squashes and cordials; some of them make some people sick and some don't.

The only liquid which is tolerated by the majority is *plain cold water*. Make sure, both at home and in hospital, that there is water at your wife's side in a glass or better still, a jug. You won't have to fight for this, just ask. No one is going to refuse a woman in labour a glass of water. Make sure it is there—and you will notice that she takes frequent small sips. No woman in labour could down half-a-pint even if she wanted to; in labour you can only take sips at frequent intervals.

In addition, it has been found that since labour is a very basic function, one's psychological needs become very basic too. And one of the basic needs a woman returns to is the need to *suck*. Pefectly mature, adult women have been discovered in labour sucking their thumbs, something they probably haven't done since they were considerably smaller! So we find that an excellent means of giving refreshment *and* satisfying this need, is to *give* her something to suck. You had better make this your special responsibility because she's almost bound to forget! Most large chemists sell off-cuts of sponges. You will find them hanging up in polythene bags near the counter where they sell the real, old-fashioned sponges. Buy her a little bag of these—they only cost a few pence each. Remember to put the sponges into her suitcase.

When you get to the hospital and are settled, ask for a saucer. Pour into it a little water from the water-jug and put the sponge in it; after a few minutes you'll have a soggy and somewhat larger sponge.

All you need to do then is pick up the sponge between every half-dozen contractions—say when the contraction finishes, squeexe it slightly so that it doesn't drip, and pass it across the lower part of her face. You'll find that, without having to be told, she will eventually reach a point when she'll suck as you pass the sponge across her mouth. Maybe you'll think "Good heavens, can't she even drink?" No, she can't—and in any case this is much more refreshing and satisfying. Here she's combining moisture and refreshment with the satisfying of a very definite need. You will notice, too, that as labour progresses, all round the outside of her lips will become very dry, almost like parchment. Make sure you keep this moist. So what with one thing and another the water in the saucer will become very murky and it will be your job to change it, too. At home, if you have a fridge, a little ice in that saucer won't do any harm either.

So (1) entertainment, (2) refreshment and (3) making sure that no one interrupts her handling of contractions—these are all your responsibilities.

Normally, human beings empty their bladder on the receipt of signals to say that it's getting full. But very often in labour one can't do this. As the baby's head descends further and further into the pelvis, the bladder gets squashed; so the normal sensory signals which indicate how full it is are often cut off. In labour, curious as this may sound, one "spends pennies" by time and not by sensation. This must be done in order to maintain the natural bladder function, to prevent it filling up and thus becoming an artificial and incidentally painful barrier to the opening cervix.

So remind her approximately once every hour to get out of bed; she's perfectly capable of doing so and I don't know of any hospital where, providing the circumstances are normal, a woman is not allowed to go to the toilet during labour. Just make sure that she goes, because she will tend to forget.

Now what if discomfort occurs as the labour progresses? Discomfort *can* occur, and it would be ridiculous to pretend that all you have to do is behave in a certain way and then there will be no pain. Sometimes there *is* considerable pain; the trick is to know what to do about it.

In normal labour the uterus itself very rarely causes pain. The pain is caused by muscles which are, so to speak, next door. It's rather like when the people next door have a bonfire in the garden—it's not your bonfire but you get the smell and the smoke. Well, during labour "smell" and "smoke" in terms of discomfort affect the muscles of the tummy, the back, and the thighs. All of you should learn our three forms of special massage for these three areas, if you haven't yet done so. It is part of the husband's job to become so familiar with these forms of massage, by practising them with his wife during labour rehearsals, that they become as natural as listening to that breathing. All three forms are both self-applicable and "slave"—applicable. (This is to make sure that your wife is not bereft of comfort if for some reason you can't be there.) You will find instructions on pages 131/3, 165/6 and 169.

So, addressing the slaves: the most valuable service of all that you can render is to give this massage if and when it is needed. All women don't need it; if they don't experience any discomfort, they won't need it and won't ask for it. But if your wife does have it, it should be caught when it is still merely mild discomfort and kept at bay. Don't wait until it's such a raging backache that she can't bear to either sit or lie, before you condescend to put down your book.

The next thing to happen is this: Suddenly you will notice, or she will tell you, that she can't handle the contraction any more. That is, when her contraction is at its height, it will no longer be enough to breathe as she has been doing. She may also tell you that she's beginning to feel pushing sensations, an intermittent pressure which is similar, but only *similar*, to the feeling when one needs to go to the lavatory and open one's bowels. Some women don't have this, but simply feel at the height of contraction what has been described as "turbulence".

Thw whole pattern of the contractions changes. And a woman trained to handle her contractions will immediately be aware of the sensation as soon as the change manifests itself. This is why she has to keep alert. Women have described how suddenly at the height of the contraction the pattern seems to go "wild"; one woman has said it was like being mixed up in a whirlpool.

However, one thing that is clear and plain is that the woman realises that she somehow can't handle it any more with Labour Diagram (3) breathing. The usual reason for this is because she has entered the *transition stage* of labour. This is the stage when most of the cervix has been taken up by the body of the uterus; but in front, just behind the pubic arch, there is still a little cervix left. So the uterus is performing a queer double function: it is still pulling up the lip of the cervix, but at the same time it is preparing for the expulsive or pushing stage of labour. This is why its action causes this peculiar sort of pattern.

Lesson 5 teaches the way of handling this stage of labour in terms of breathing, position, and control. What you must do is recognise that this stage of labour is the most difficult stage to handle. This is not because the contractions are longer or stronger; on the contrary, they are frequently shorter and weaker. It is because there is a distinct *emotional* change, a change which is as inevitable as the fact that the baby will later be born. In fact, all through this labour, you will be aware of all sorts of emotional changes—the wild excitement at the beginning, the feeling of "aren't-I-clever" smugness peculiar to trained women when they first have Labour Diagram (2) contractions and have to go into Level C to breathe for comfort, the look of almost holy concentration when the contractions become stronger and they have their work cut out to keep up with them. This is an equally typical change which occurs at the transition stage.

The change will be one of two kinds; as you will once again be the victim, you might as well know now what these are! With the first kind, the woman suddenly becomes terribly tired and sleepy. Whether she's been in labour two hours or twelve doesn't seem to make any difference. She suddenly says, "If only I could just shut my eyes between contractions." This is of course the one thing she must *not* do. It will reduce her alertness. So your job will be to encourage her, persuade her, even blackmail her into keeping awake!

The other alternative is, that she will become, and this is the only word I can use, an irritable, nasty-tempered shrew. Yes, even your charming, delightful wife. Suddenly, the kind things you've been doing for her until now—massaging, giving her drinks and sips of the sponge—all these things that have earned you a grateful "thank-you, darling" will be meaningless. All of a sudden, nothing you can do will be right. You'll be doing the wrong thing *whatever* you do. Now remember that this is an emotional change which *she can't control*. She's not being deliberately nasty. If you have married a very sweet girl, and you have never known her to be anything but sweet, don't be too shocked, either. She may use swear-words you never even thought she knew!

The nicest people sometimes have the most violent emotional change. On page 118 you will find my account of the charming little Japanese girl who could speak no English but who managed to understand my instructions with the help of her English-speaking husband during labour. She was alone with me during transition stage and suddenly said "I do not hear Engliss, now!" That was Oriental perversity; but I wanted to laugh because it provided such a perfect universal example! As soon as her second stage of labour started she became a sweet girl again, but until that moment she wouldn't have anything to do with me.

The only way out of transition stage is through it; this of course is the emotion that makes life difficult for everybody. Here your support becomes invaluable. First, because you may have to verbally establish the rhythm of breathing with each contraction, as you did during labour rehearsals, over and over and over again. Second, it becomes a very important "anchor", as one woman has described it, to hear the voice.

Something else which is of tremendous value is what is called, for want of a better term, *physical contact*. This is what to do. If she becomes very restless, put your hand very lightly on her wrist and keep it there. When the contraction becomes stronger and the turbulence more marked, increase the pressure on the wrist until you've got her in a very firm grip, as though she were an escaping prisoner. Keep this grip hard until the contraction becomes weaker again—you will know by the way her breathing changes. Then gradually release your hold until at the end of the contraction you end up with your hand lightly on her wrist again.

Now some women don't like this. They really feel as if they were being imprisoned. You will be left in absolutely no doubt as to whether she likes it or not! If she hates this pressure on her wrist, do it on her shoulder. She won't object and it will be almost as good in effect. Don't allow her to *hold* your hand. There is a temptation when you hold someone's fingers to squeeze them and this means she will be contracting her hand. That's why it has to be wrist or shoulder, not "Hold tightly on to my hand, my love"—that went out with the Victorians. We want to relax those muscles, not tighten them.

To summarise then: physical contact, verbal reiteration of command and DON'T for heaven's sake argue with her should she become bad tempered, and DON'T try to make her reasonable. She just *can't* be reasonable. If she wants to have a little cry, encourage her. It releases nervous tension and is part of the cycle.

One more thing you *must* do. When she gets to this stage and it's quite obvious she's there, you must let the midwife know. If it's a home confinement, the midwife has already been once, gone and not yet returned, now is the time to let her know. In hospital you ring the bell. When someone comes, don't say "I think my wife is in transition stage". The accepted phrase is "I think my wife is going to need to push soon." And it is indeed the literal truth.

Whoever it is will pull back the bedclothes and observe the external surface of the pelvic floor, which of course is visible as soon as the legs are extended. You may wonder, what on earth is being looked at, what do they hope to see? Well, if you are both right, at the height of the next contraction they will see a slight movement of the walls of the vagina as the baby's head begins to establish itself in the birth canal. This is what they're waiting for. If everyone agrees that you're right, the next thing to happen is that your wife will be transported by wheel-chair or trolley to the labour ward, second stage room, delivery room, or whatever it is called.

And here let me give you a good tip—and a *real* chance to play Sir Galahad. Even if your particular hospital has previously said they will only allow husbands in during the first stage of labour but not the second, try and make another bid. You haven't anything to lose, have you? What you do is this: attach yourself to the trolley or wheel chair and just go with it! There's no point in saying "Excuse me, but would you mind if I came too?" Just go of your own accord. Now in the hurry and bustle of a large hospital—you know, these hospitals which cover areas where the whole of a new town is involved—you can do this quite easily, because there are lots of people around anyway.

If you get to the labour ward and no one has noticed and asked you what the devil you're doing—so far so good. But now you have to be very careful. You have to watch what everyone else does and do it too. By pure mimicry! They will all be putting on their white gowns. May I remind you that this white gown fastens at the back? You see if you get to this point and then put it on like an ordinary coat, all is lost! Just look as though you belonged. And watch.

If everyone else is putting on a mask, you do the same. (Usually it's in a little container, and often disposable, with two loops to fit over the ears.) If no one else does, neither do you. Just stay with it and *just belong*. As soon as you look awkward and out of place, you will be noticed. I know two London hospitals at least that now allow husbands in the second-stage room as a matter of course, thanks to the audacity and courage of two men who first made it in this way!

Of course you may be caught red-handed. Well, you won't have lost anything, and it's worth trying, even if you do end up pacing the floor with the others.

When you do make it, your place is on your wife's left

Diagram 26 Before labour begins

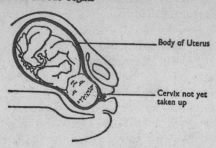

Body of Uterus

Cervix not yet
taken up

Diagram 27 Pre-labour phase

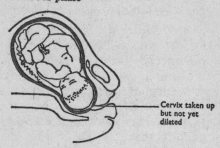

Cervix taken up
but not yet
dilated

Diagram 28 End of the first stage

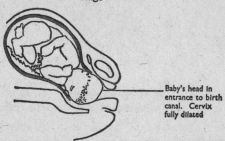

Baby's head in
entrance to birth
canal. Cervix
fully dilated

side, near her head and shoulders. And your job is as follows:

(1) Continue to encourage her in handling her contractions with transition stage breathing.

(2) Do so until either (a) the urge to push becomes completely irresistible, in which case—whatever you do or whatever anyone else says—she will make a pushing effort because she can't help it; this is physiologically quite correct; or (b) the midwife or doctor will say "You can push now, I can see the baby's head". They don't mean this in quite the sense you may think. What in fact they mean is that at the height of the contraction a little of the crown of the baby's head is just visible.

Either (a) or (b) indicates that we have entered the second or expulsive stage of labour. Then your job is as follows:

(3) Support her in expulsive drill, which by then should be as familiar to you as Level A breathing. Support the leg on your side at the calf, so that you take the weight. And also

(4) Help to keep her head forward on her chest, while she is blocking her breathing and pushing.

You will then have the fascinating experience of seeing more and more of the baby's head with each contraction; you will notice that at the height of the contraction it comes down more, and as the contraction weakens and goes away, it apparently goes back again. Actually it doesn't really do this. Correctly handled, it moves three steps forward and half a step back. (Incorrectly handled it's three steps forward and two-and-a-half steps back, so you can see why the expulsive stage of labour is much more efficient and much faster with our method.)

Gradually more and more of the baby's head will emerge, until you get to the point when it "crowns". Crowning means exactly that—the crown of the baby's head is visible outside the mother's body. Then we know that the next contraction will deliver the baby's head to below the chin. The baby's chin will be nearest to the mother's back passage. For this contraction she will be told to stop pushing, so that the uterus can deliver the baby's head slowly and gently. You will then see something very interesting: the baby turns round. It does this all by itself but with the midwife just supporting it. Which way it turns depends on the position it had in the uterus; it does this so that the shoulders can be delivered one by one and so make its passage easier.

So with the next contraction you will see first, the front shoulder and arm emerge from the mother's body, then the next shoulder and arm. The remainder of the baby slides out without any effort, or certainly without any conscious effort. This is the end of the second or expulsive stage of labour and the baby is now born.

You will observe that your baby will be a very odd colour, a strange sort of blue-grey-mauve mixture. When it begins to cry, sometime between the moment when its head emerges and the rest of its body arrives, then it will take on the familiar vivid, bright pink colour of new-born babies. This colour is different from that of your skin or mine, because such a colour comes after exposure to the air for some time. By the way, the cry that a new-born baby makes does not indicate pain. It indicates the first conscious, deliberate inflating of the lungs.

You will also notice the umbilical cord, looking like a thickened version of the vein in your wrist, and about the same colour too. This still goes in through the vagina, as it is attached to the placenta which is still in the uterus.

From the moment the baby is born, the third stage of labour has begun and fortunately you don't have anything

Diagram 29   The second stage

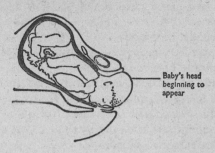

Baby's head
beginning to
appear

Diagram 30

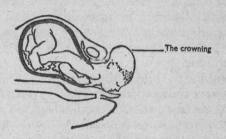

The crowning

Diagram 31

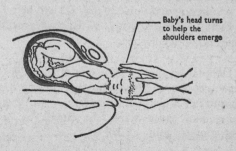

Baby's head turns
to help the
shoulders emerge

to do. If you watch, you will see the cord clipped, usually with two metal clips acting as tourniquets, and then cut between the two clips. Then the baby is fully independent—at last!

It will be wrapped in a warm towel, sheet or whatever, and should be given to your wife to hold in her arms. I say "should" because sometimes there are medical reasons why it needs to have some attention first; but at other times this merely seems to be forgotten. A simple "Could I hold my baby a minute?" will remedy this—unless of course there *are* medical reasons against it.

You may also notice that while the baby is still lying on the bed, the midwife will put a rubber tube into its mouth, then take the other end of the tube in her own mouth and suck. This is to clear the passages of mucus and help the baby to breathe. In some hospitals it's a completely standard procedure with every baby, so it's nothing to worry about. And it doesn't bother either the baby or the person doing it!

Withing 10 to 15 minutes the placenta separates; usually one more contraction will deliver it, with a little assistance from the mother. And that completes labour. All that usually happens subsequently is that the mother is cleaned up a little. She will be bleeding rather as she does during a heavy period, so she is given sanitary protection.

If you are faced with the delivery of your child with no qualified assistance available because labour is so rapid, I will tell you what you can do that will be perfectly safe.

First, reassure your wife—this can be a somewhat frightening experience.

DON'T try any fancy obstetric tricks. This particular baby will get itself born quite well, as it has already got this far and needs no assistance from you. Your wife, however, does need your help. She needs to be reassured that everything is going well.

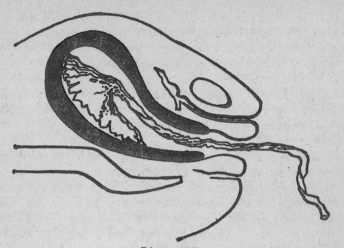

Diagram 32
The third stage of labour: Uterus contracts as placenta separates

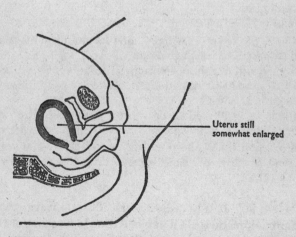

Uterus still somewhat enlarged

Diagram 33
Pelvic Basin after the end of labour

If you can see the baby's head *DO remind her not to push*. This baby is probably getting itself born without any mechanical assistance from her tummy muscles. As soon as the baby is born it will probably yell lustily.

DON'T try to tie the cord, nor to clip or cut it.

Make sure the baby's mouth has no mucus inside. If it has, just put a finger in and get it out.

DO cover the baby up. It has lived at body temperature for nine months and this is not body temperature now. Anything will do—a blanket, overcoat or jacket. Make sure too, that your wife is covered as the same applies to her: she will be hot, for labour is an energy-producing activity. Now, suddenly, there is a phsyiological anti-climax, and she needs to be kept warm.

You will find that the placenta will probably follow almost immediately. Cover the placenta with some newspaper—just for aesthetic reasons.

DON'T try to separate baby and placenta, and make sure that the baby's face isn't covered.

Then go and telephone—either the ambulance if you were going to go to hospital and didn't make it, or the midwife if she was coming.

This is all you need to do—and it is actually the safest kind of delivery. It doesn't need any mechanical assistance; the more you fiddle about and try to think of what you've seen on T.V., the more dangerous you're likely to be to your wife and child!

WARNING: It is actually illegal, if it can be proved, to *not* summon medical aid if you had time to do so before this event. It's just not worth the risk—and doctors and midwives *do* know what they're doing, whatever you may think.

One final thing to do when you have tidied up and made your phone call: put on the kettle and make a cup of tea. You will *both* need one! In hospital, of course, the eternal cuppa will appear automatically at this moment. And how welcome it is!

But personally I often feel a twinge of nostalgia for the first time I ever attended a delivery in a French hospital. When it was all over, the Matron bore me off to her room; going to a large cupboard in the corner she remarked to me, "What will you have?" I could hardly believe my ears! But sure enough, we all had brandies or whiskies or whatever— including the mother and father. Ah well—the British will insist on remaining individualists, whatever the situation ...

MEMO TO MOTHERS AND MIDWIVES

Lifting the "curse"

HOW many women there must be who from earliest girlhood are plagued with painful periods. The colloquial name "curse" is surely a clear indication. Theories have been produced over the years about the reasons for this but very few practical answers have been found. I was actually *forced* to think about this problem.

One day a doctor telephoned me. He said he had a patient, a young girl of 17, who was having such painful periods that he had to give her ever-increasing doses of drugs just to make life bearable for her during her monthly rhythm. This doctor's appeal was a real cry of despair because no matter what he tried everything lost its value after a little while. He thought that I, who had mastered the problem of pain in labour, might be able to come up with something.

From this "emergency" a syllabus developed for teaching girls and women how to subdue the painful part of their period. Several nurses up and down the country have used it with good results. Any woman can teach it to her friend or her teenage daughter; my small daughter of 11 has taught it in a simplified form to some of her friends. Most important is the fact that any woman who has learnt to handle her labour can, if she needs to, use these simple rules during her own menstrual cycle.

It might be necessary to point out to you that if the patient is a very young girl, you should not mention that the exercises for "curse" pains are those which are taught to expectant mothers! On the other hand, several of my young girl patients have remarked "If this helps me during a period isn't it possible that it might also help me when I have a baby?"

This of course gave me a splendid opportunity to "come clean" and to discuss with them what you have just read in this book. I hope it will do a little to save these girls unnecessary fear about something which can, if correctly handled, be such a wonderful experience.

I have divided the course into lessons just like the course for labour.

Lesson 1: "The story of reproduction" as in Lesson 2 but without reference to conception and pregnancy. Practical work: active decontraction-drill and Level A breathing, as in Lesson 1.

Lesson 2: Check practical work from previous lesson. Teach Level B and Level C breathing plus disassociation-drill as in Lesson 3.

Lesson 3: Check each level of disassociation-drill and combine it with breathing as in Labour Diagram (2).

Lesson 4: Check Disassociation-drill with conscious controlled breathing, as learnt in Lesson 3, and teach "dry land swimming". Find a pouffe or a low coffee-table and put a pillow on top for comfort. Make your pupil lie on this on her tummy and support herself with her hands on the floor. Then teach her to kick her legs—the way she would if she were swimming breast-stroke. This movement should be done rhythmically and continued for about two minutes.

Instructions for monthly routine

Once the exercises are semi-automatic, the pupil should go over them again three or four times during the last half of her monthly cycle. In the last ten days before her next period is due, she should do "dry land swimming" every day for about six minutes, in two-minute bouts. (This helps to relieve pelvic congestion.)

When the discomfort of her period begins, a pleasantly warm bath will be very comforting. It should be followed by going to bed with a hot-water bottle tucked against the small of the back; lying in the "basic position" (Lesson 1) she should handle the pain as a Labour Diagram (2) contraction, which is what it really is.

During the first monthly period after the four lessons your pupil will discover that the pain is not continuous but wavelike, with intervals of rest in between. This will seem new to her because her previous tension will not have allowed her to become aware of this.

Each month for about six months have your pupil report, by phone if you like, how she has handled each period. All sorts of changes from previous patterns are common. Irregular periods tend to become more regular; the pain-phase of each period is much reduced in length and intensity.

Finally most pupils can handle what is left without the bath/bed routine but just with an hour sitting in a chair when they are able to quietly concentrate. The lessening of the overwhelming fatigue from which so many women suffer is also very noticeable.

Drugs should *not* be used at the same time as this routine is followed.

I hope that you will feel with me that this drill is a real weapon to combat the "curse" which women have carried with them for far too long.

POSTSCRIPT FOR PROFESSIONALS

To all workers in the field of
ante-natal care

I sincerely hope that the way in which this book is written has not annoyed you.

I have deliberately spoken to the mother directly because even experienced doctors, midwives and physiotherapists often find it difficult to convert professional language into simple terms; and these *are* needed to clarify what mothers often overhear but only half-understand.

It is also unfortunately true that one's clinical and theoretical knowledge does not necessarily make one able to communicate the essence of such knowledge to others. So I have used the ordinary words and phrases which I use in my daily classes for mothers. I have found that this helps mothers to understand what they can do during labour and to understand in general what you might do, too. From your point of view, this book could therefore be a useful basis on which to build your own talks and classes for expectant mothers.

For reason of greater visual clarity, scientific accuracy has had to be sacrificed in the anatomical diagrams.

The index at the end may also help you in collecting teaching-aids to clarify your words and amplify the expression of your ideas.

Perhaps you do not actually teach expectant mothers but meet them in the labour ward. In that case I hope that this book will be the means of clarifying what trained mothers have been taught, and that you will be able to support them with *your* understanding of the principles they have been taught. A trained mother does not need someone to sit with her during every moment of labour. She should, however, be able to have her husband's companionship if desired, as well as the security of knowing that a member of the labour ward staff will be able to strengthen her control by reminding her if necessary of her training.

If you are interested in any further technical background to the psychoprophylactic method, you may like to know that there are special seminars for professional workers in the maternity field. Detailed information about them, and appropriate dates, can be obtained from the organisation whose name and address I give below. The people there will welcome any queries from you; they too are anxious to put the tools of high level ante-natal preparation into the hands of people who care for expectant mothers. You should write to:

The National Childbirth Trust,
9 Queensborough Terrace,
Bayswater,
London W2 3TB

ERNA WRIGHT

INDEX

Teaching aids, films, books and pamphlets, accessories

TEACHING AIDS:

Chiltern "Lullaby" Baby-Doll. This doll has a soft cloth body filled with foam rubber chippings and plastic arms and legs. 13 ins. long, (obtainable from most good toy-shops).

New-born Baby Doll. This is a doll which weighs $6\frac{1}{4}$ lbs., is 20 ins. long and has a head-circumference of $13\frac{3}{4}$ ins. Made on the "Bendy-toy" principle to show flexion of limbs in the new-born baby. Useful for showing expectant mothers how large their baby might be at birth. Price on application from Educational & Scientific Plastics, Holmthorpe Avenue, Redhill, Surrey.

Plastic Pelvis. Educational & Scientific Plastics; address as above. Price on application from Educational & Scientific Plastics.

Birth-Atlas. Very large, suitable for a class of 10–15 mothers to see clearly. Price on application from H. K. Lewis & Co., 136 Gower Street, London, W.C.1.

"A Baby is Born". A smaller edition of the Birth Atlas but more comprehensive and with more diagrams. Also translations in French, German and Spanish. Suitable for 3–4 mothers to see clearly. Price on application from H. K. Lewis & Co. at the above address.

Note: There may be a six-week wait for this publication.

Taki-Bak (a washable, transparent covering suitable for the above charts). You should send a stamped addressed envelope to The National Childbirth Trust, 9 Queensborough Terrace, Bayswater, London W2 3TB.

"Birthday Slides"—taken from the film "Birthday". 20 slides in colour showing diagrams of conception and growth of the foetus, illustrations of the positions of the baby's head as it descends and passes through the birth canal; 10 black-and-white slides of an actual birth. From The National Childbirth Trust, 9 Queensborough Terrace, Bayswater, London W2 3TB. Price £5.25, includes postage (inland).

FILMS

"Birthday" made by Messrs. Smith, Kline & French, Welwyn Garden City, Herts. Shows the training of six expectant mothers, using the principles of psychoprophylaxis, and the birth of two of the "class" babies. Very useful for showing to a group of mothers who have almost completed their course of training according to these principles. (*Not* useful for showing to mothers who are attending relaxation classes.) The film is 16 mm. colour and sound; it may be borrowed from The National Childbirth Trust, 9 Queensborough Terrace, Bayswater, London W2 3TB. Cost of hiring £3.50 + VAT per showing. Applications should be made 6–8 weeks in advance upon written application by a *bone fide* teacher.

Note: there is a waiting list because the film is very much in demand so book 6–8 weeks in advance of need.

A Family Affair. (Birth, Growth and Development, Pt. 1.) A 15 min. 16 mm. silent film in black-and-white, with captions. A written commentary is supplied. This charming film, made by students at Birmingham Teachers Training College, shows the birth of a trained mother's third baby. It shows some ante-natal preparation and the birth of the baby in the mother's own home. It is filmed over the mother's shoulder to give the mother's own view of the birth. The film shows the effect of a new baby's arrival within the family unit. It is admirably suited for showing as an introduction to the idea of training to all types of audience, including teenagers. From Leonard Ellis Ltd., 23 Bristol Road, Birmingham 5. Price £1 per showing.

Books

Babies without Tears. By Marjorie Karmel. Secker & Warburg (1959). A personal experience of psychoprophylaxis as a patient of Dr. Lamaze in France plus the author's account of her attempts to introduce these ideas to her doctor in the U.S.A. Very readable, price £1.50.

The First Nine Months of Life. By Geraldine Lux Flanagan. From most good bookshops. Price 90p. Heinemann Medical Books Ltd.

Baby and Child Care. By Dr. Benjamin Spock. This charming book has become a classic in its field and should be in the hands of every woman who is expecting a baby. British paper-back edition published by New English Library. Price $52\frac{1}{2}$p.

Leaflets and Booklets

Easier Childbirth. By Elliot Philipp, f.r.c.s., f.r.c.o.g., and Ruth Forbes, j.p., s.c.m. Published by the B.M.A., a booklet of introduction to the use of psychoprophylaxis in childbirth. Available from Boots and all good Chemists. Price 10p.

Easy Breastfeeding. A comprehensive leaflet written by a midwife who made the feeding of young babies her special subject. Published by and obtainable from National Childbirth Trust, 9 Queensborough Terrace, Bayswater, London W2 3TB, Price 10p. Please include a stamped addressed envelope.

Your Baby and Your Figure. By the Obstetric Association of Chartered Physiotherapists. A very clear and simple description of the few important post-natal exercises. Published by Livingstone (1961). Price 15p.

Brassieres for Pregnancy and Breastfeeding

MAVA Brassiere. All new mothers want to look pretty and feel comfortable. The Mava Bra is the ideal garment to help them.

Bust measurements increase unpredictably during pregnancy and in the first days of lactation. The usual nursing bra is inadequately designed to cope with this.

The Mava has the following excellent features:

Back lacing which allows the bra to enlarge with the breasts.

Adjustable shoulder straps.

Deep cut waistline, which gives firm support underneath. With the adjustable straps this obviates the need for different cup sizes.

Front opening for nursing, with a safety strap to stop the bra slipping.

Sizes: Mava is made in sizes increasing every inch from 32–40 ins. and every two inches from 40–44 ins. There are several different cup-fittings in addition to the usual commercial ones.

Available only from The National Childbirth Trust, 9 Queensborough Terrace, London W2 3TB. Send a stamped addressed envelope and ask for full details of price and order form to ensure correct self-fitting by post. Personal fittings by appointment only.

It is necessary that the lacing of the bra should meet during pregnancy, but during the first two weeks of lactation it is usual to have a gap of about one inch. Ideally, Mava bras should be bought at about 28–30 weeks pregnancy and can then be worn for the remainder of the pregnancy and during lactation.

Glossary of Terms

Lesson Notes